August 1997

50
7-00

You've been a wonderful husband.
You'll be a wonderful father too.

HOW TO
I love you

PAMPER
YOUR
PREGNANT
WIFE

by

Ron Schultz and Sam Schultz

D1446895

 **Meadowbrook Press**
Distributed by Simon & Schuster
New York

Library of Congress Cataloging-in-Publication Data

Schultz, Ron, 1951-
    How to pamper your pregnant wife / by Ron Schultz
    and Sam Schultz.
        p.   cm.
    Includes bibliographical references.
    ISBN 0-88166-269-0 (Meadowbrook).
    ISBN 0-671-57495-7 (Simon & Schuster)
        1. Pregnancy. 2. Childbirth. 3. Husbands. 4. Fathers.
    I. Schultz, Sam, 1921-   . II. Title.
    RG525.S393   1997
    618.2'4--dc21   96-45212
                                           CIP

Editor: Liya Lev Oertel
Copyeditor: Nancy Baldrica
Production Manager: Amy Unger
Desktop Publishing Manager: Danielle White
Text and Cover Design: MacLean & Tuminelly

Text © 1996 by Ron Schultz and Sam Schultz

Cover photo © 1990 Michael Norton/Adstock

Published by Meadowbrook Press, 5451 Smetana Drive,
Minnetonka, MN 55343.

BOOK TRADE DISTRIBUTION by Simon & Schuster, a divi-
sion of Simon and Schuster, Inc., 1230 Avenue of the
Americas, New York, NY 10020.

00 99 98 97   10 9 8 7 6 5 4 3 2 1

Printed in the United States of America.

ACKNOWLEDGEMENTS

We would like to thank the following people for their help in preparing this book: Dr. Stephen V. Lieb, Tara Fellner, Laura Sanderford, Marvin Klotz, Peggy Aylsworth, Christie Romero, and the editorial staff at Meadowbrook Press, especially Bruce Lansky who knew we had something with this book. A special thanks to all the pregnant husbands and wives who so willingly told us their honest and often intimate stories about their pregnancies.

This book is dedicated to
soon-to-be fathers, everywhere.
May you find the same joy
we have found in our children.

TABLE OF CONTENTS

Introduction...**3**

What Is Pampering?..**5**

First Trimester..**9**

Discovering You're Pregnant **9**
Outlasting Morning Sickness.....................................**10**
Will Life Ever Be the Same? **12**
What Happened to My Waistline?..............................**16**
Weathering the Sudden Mood Shifts, or—
    Yes, Dear. I'm with You All the Way **17**
Changing Lifestyles **18**
An Unmentionable—Miscarriage **22**
More Changes **23**
To Read or Not to Read? Buying Pregnancy Books **25**
Eating Properly...**26**
Talking to the Baby **28**
Sex and the Pregnant Wife **29**
Congratulations! You've Made It through
    the First Trimester...**31**
Keeping Her Happy..**33**

Second Trimester..**35**

Say Good-Bye to Morning Sickness **35**
You're Not Fat, You're Pregnant................................**36**
What to Wear? **39**
Helping Her through the Amniocentesis **40**
In-Laws Don't Have to Be Out-Laws **43**
Telling the World You're Pregnant.............................**45**
Folklore Is for Reading—
    Not Necessarily for Following...............................**46**
Some Of Our Favorite Superstitions about Pregnancy **47**
Yesterday and Today..**48**
Naming the Baby...**49**

More Sex and the Pregnant Wife 52
No, That's Not a Stretch Mark! **56**
Exercising Your Pregnant Wife **58**
The Grazing Goes On **60**
You Deserve to Feel Good about Yourself **61**
Keeping Her Happy **62**

Third Trimester **65**

Of Course, I Still Love You **65**
Building the Nest...Again **66**
Do Your Shopping Early **68**
Getting Ready for the Birth—
   Take a Cleansing Breath **70**
Checking Out the Hospital **73**
Still More Sex and the Pregnant Wife **75**
Getting Ready for the Trip to the Hospital **76**
The Birthing Choice—Whose Decision Is It? **77**
Discussing Hospital Procedures with Your OB/GYN **80**
The Last Weeks **81**
Learning How Far You Can Go from Your Wife **83**
Traveling Away from Home **85**
Soothing the Anxious Wife **86**
More Superstitions **87**
The Night Before **88**
Timing Contractions **89**
Delivery Dad's Obligations **90**
What's Been Going On inside Your Wife's Body
   during the Third Trimester? **92**
Checking into the Hospital **93**
Getting into Your Room **93**
So, What's Happening to My Wife **96**
Keeping Her Happy **98**
You Made It, Didn't You? **99**

Letter from a Pampered Wife (Ron's) **100**
Bibliography **101**

INTRODUCTION

S o, she's pregnant. Congratulations! A baby, a tike, an heir apparent. Welcome to the club, Dad! Now you've got nine full months, or so, to focus on making the leap from that free-spirited attitude you had before attaining fatherhood (when you were able to do what you wanted when you wanted) to being a caring, loving, responsible father. Really, though, you're going to be fine. And if you follow the helpful advice in this book, so, too, will your wife.

Why? Because *How to Pamper Your Pregnant Wife* is about relationships and feelings—*not* about overburdening clinical information that can make pregnancy seem too clinical. Nonetheless, we will do our best to make you cognizant of what you should be aware and why. You'll also find here some pertinent medical and scientific facts (in capsulized form) obtained from pediatricians, obstetricians/gynecologists (OB/GYNs), and psychologists. And we'll include a smattering of homespun suggestions garnered through interviews, research, and actual experiences that relate to what a man gets into after his wife gets pregnant.

We don't pretend to speak as professionals—we speak from a layman's point of view, and as once-concerned pregnant fathers ourselves, who realize it takes two to tango, and who know there's an easy and most rewarding way to finish the dance.

Actually, a lot of the things we'll cover come intuitively to soon-to-be fathers. We hope the information in this book will help bring out your instinctive nature and help you discover what, in many cases, you already know. And we hope to do it with compassion. You'll find that this book is filled with advice, rules, suggestions, guidelines, buzzwords (loving words to say to her), and other relevant and comforting information. All of these thoughts were volunteered by fellow fathers who supported and pampered their wives through the heart-felt wonders and perils of pregnancy. We also conducted dozens of interviews with pregnant wives, doctors, lawyers, therapists, mothers-in-law, mothers, marriage and family counselors, and even children who remember events that led up to the birth of their siblings. Their feelings, experiences, and expertise will also be reflected in this book.

WHAT IS PAMPERING?

Pampering is more than just hugging and kissing. That's not enough for a pregnant wife. She needs and deserves a lot more, and only you can provide it. Pampering is consideration—showing you care in little ways, such as going with her for check-ups, not always, but once in a while. Pampering is support—for example, listening, not answering, when she might be scared or demanding. Pampering is love—the connection that brought you two here in the first place.

Now, onward into the fray. Remember, your wife can't get any more pregnant than she already is. And you can't overdo showering her with consideration, support, and love.

To help you along, the first thing you must come to terms with, Dad, is that contrary to any of the physical laws and forces of nature you may have heard about, you're pregnant, too! Before you take exception to that remark, consider this— isn't it true that today's fathers, like you, are more sensitive, caring men? True. They're more understanding and sympathetic toward their wives during pregnancy? True. They find themselves wanting to become more intently and intimately involved in every aspect of the pregnancy? True. So since you're going through what she's going through, YOU'RE PREGNANT, TOO! True? True!

No need to panic. No need to feel defensive. Yours is not an isolated case. This year alone there will be nearly 30 million pregnant fathers in India, 19 million pregnant fathers in China, 6 million pregnant fathers in the former Soviet Union, and 4 million pregnant fathers in the USA. According to Britannica World Data, this year there will be more than 145 million pregnant fathers worldwide. That's more fathers than play soccer,

5

basketball, pool, football, cricket, baseball, golf, and bocci combined. Well, maybe not bocci. To give you a better idea of how many pregnant fathers there are every year, here's a bit of interesting trivia—every four seconds, every day of the year, somewhere in this world, a woman gives birth to a baby.

But don't think that makes your pregnancy any less unique. For you and yours it is and could be a very special celebration—if you choose to make it that way.

What you will find in the pages to come, then, is a trimester-by-trimester crash course in pregnant relations (trimesters are the basic three-month periods by which a human pregnancy is divided). If you thought getting married required some adjustment on your part, well, be prepared to readjust some more. This is not to imply you won't love being pregnant with your wife. The popular consensus, according to 99.6 percent of the pregnant fathers we interviewed, is that having a baby is one of the most rewarding and gratifying experiences of their lives. Really! Getting there, however, may mean that you will have to throw many of your typically male preconceptions of logical adult behavior out the window. Logic has no place in the baby-making game—it didn't at the time of conception, and you shouldn't expect it now.

It's common knowledge that pregnant fathers often experience a myriad of anxieties, doubts, and apprehensions. Not unusual. That's a positive sign that changes are about to take place. Anxiety is up, energy is down, and any logical thinking man with an iota of sensitivity coursing through his veins will realize that compromise and understanding must now become the order of the day. That's not easy for some men to accept. But you can accept this: it's not unmanly to exhibit delight at the prospect of becoming a father. What's more, your delight will certainly reassure your wife that you're as excited about the pregnancy as she is.

Now, you may have heard all those "good buddy" remarks

about how you'll just have to suffer through it. Not true! We're going to show you the joy in this process, and in so doing, we're going to also help you appreciate your wife's pregnancy. After all, she will, in all probability, suffer far more than you will. Trust us, she'll need lots of pampering.

You see, up until that potent "moment of truth," when the two of you took a dive into the gene pool, your wife probably functioned at her normal hormonal balance. Now, it's a whole new ball game. Within hours of your fateful coupling, millions of little hormone hotrods poured out into her system. Their job is to create a new chemical balance in your wife's system. Of course, this new body chemistry initially creates a chemical and emotional imbalance inside your wife that roller coasters her moods from high to low in a matter of seconds. All pregnant women experience it. It goes with the territory. Your wife can be laughing one moment and crying the next moment. Those hormones affect your wife's sex drive as well as her behavior. They can also affect her energy, leaving her completely exhausted or uncommonly energized at day's end. The main culprits are estrogen and progesterone: They bombard your wife's body in greater quantities than ever before. But the good thing about those ever-present fluctuating-in-intensity creatures is that they prime your wife's body to sustain the delicate fetus.

You may need a lot of understanding to be able to cope with your wife's hormonal mood swings, but the end result is worth every anxious moment you may experience. So the next time your wife goes through one of her emotional swings, what could be nicer than holding her, stroking her, and making sure she knows that you understand the upheaval that's going on inside her? If you can do that, you can help make this pregnancy a truly remarkable experience for both of you. Your wife will appreciate your pampering.

FIRST TRIMESTER

Discovering You're Pregnant

Fathers find out they're pregnant in as many ways as there are pregnancies. One father we spoke to told us about that first special occasion when the contraceptives were, purposely, left in the drawer. The next morning, after what he hoped would be the first of many romantically planned evenings filled with lovemaking, his wife insisted she was pregnant. The first morning after! As it turned out, she was right. It should be added that he told us, with a mischievous grin, that after a few days of mental and emotional adjustment, they eventually continued with his original plan.

Nature's surefire warning sign that something is stirring is, of course, the missed period. Where once you may have prayerfully counted the days for that cleansing flow to arrive, you may now find yourselves praying intensely for a "no flow."

Once your wife is a week or so late, it's usually time to play doctor. You rush out to buy a home pregnancy test to check some of that first-morning pee. Then comes the agonizing wait. Does the doughnut ring appear in the tube? Does the color change, the plus sign show up? Are you too early? Is there something wrong with the test? Maybe you somehow mixed up your pee with hers. The waiting is nerve-racking.

The real test comes a week or so later when you and your wife see her OB/GYN. Yes, you get to go, too. In fact, you should plan to go with her to many of her prenatal visits. It's a pampering way to let her know that you're concerned, and that she has your full support.

Some husbands may find that on these initial visits to the OB/GYN, their wives experience some denial. We know of one wife who insisted, after her results came back positive, that she wasn't pregnant. She just knew it was gas. This went on and on. Her understanding husband, knowing full well they were quite pregnant, gently pampered her through the transition by agreeing with her and insisting they continue to see her doctor for the sake of her health. He told us that his wife maintained her denial until the baby was born, when she said rather sheepishly, "I guess it wasn't gas after all." Patience, Dad. You may need plenty of gentle reassurance and a profusion of patience.

Outlasting Morning Sickness

Another sure sign of pregnancy is the misnomer known as "morning sickness." If your wife spends a good part of the day and night worshipping at the altar of the porcelain gods, there's good reason. It's due to the massive hormonal influx your wife is experiencing and has absolutely nothing to do with the chicken, lobster, or arugula she ate the night before. Morning sickness is a very positive sign that the pregnancy is in good shape. It tells you those hormones are doing their thing. Admittedly, however, it takes a special kind of woman to be able to say through the nausea and vomiting, "I'm so happy I'm pregnant."

Morning sickness was an ongoing occurrence in my household. (When we refer to ourselves in the first person, we are talking about Ron. Unless, of course, we are talking about Sam, Ron's father.) I have always done the cooking at home. My wife's culinary abilities are limited to turning on the microwave, slicing a piece of fruit, or fixing an instant breakfast. Fortunately for us, I enjoy cooking. After all, how many nights a week can two happily married people have instant breakfast together and remain happily married?

Each morning when we would awaken, I would nudge close to my wonderfully blossoming beloved, rub her tummy, and cheerfully ask, "What would you like to throw up this morning, dear?" Fortunately for me, my wife has a great sense of humor. Unfortunately for her, breakfast had to be served in two shifts. The first would be sacrificed to the gods. The second (the one that usually stayed down) would be anything she could tolerate. On the days she couldn't tolerate any food at all, her sense of humor was sorely lacking. So I'd rub her back, kiss her on the forehead, and comfort her as best I could. Comforting and loving words would help. And depending on her disposition, I'd ask her what, in her wildest fantasy, she might crave. If it wasn't in the house, and if it was obtainable, I'd make an effort to go out and get it for her. She'd usually stop me before I left, because she'd changed her mind, but just offering to do it made her feel better.

We have also recorded a number of stories from fathers who experienced times of morning sickness themselves. The clinical term is Couvade Syndrome—from the French "to brood or hatch." Psychologists have referred to it as "man's defensive mechanism at work." To compensate for his wife's suffering, a husband takes on his wife's patterns of distress, such as nausea, food cravings, and even weight gain.

The rush for the bathroom in those homes is always a perilous undertaking. These sympathetic signs of pregnancy were not uncommon in our house. I felt nauseous the first couple of weeks of our pregnancy, until my wife started getting sick. Then, my sickness went away. She still insists she was acting sick for my sake. Sometimes dads need pampering, too. (Wives know that.) An important point to remember, however, is if you're both sick together, she always has the right of way.

What is the best way to deal with your wife when her system is doing the fantastic flip-flop? A good piece of advice is to hold the advice. As well meaning as it may be, your advice probably will not be well received. The better part of valor is to allow your wife some privacy. Our interviews reveal that most pregnant wives prefer a little solitude at these rather awkward moments. That doesn't mean you can't shout out a few comforting words from the other side of the door—or, maybe, apply a cool compress to the back of her neck. These are usually the most effective ways to handle the situation. Thankfully, most bouts with morning sickness miraculously disappear at the beginning of the second trimester. But, in the middle of it all, a genuinely empathetic, "Oh, honey, I'm so sorry," is usually a safe bet.

Will Life Ever Be the Same?

With all these sudden and dramatic changes sweeping into your lives, you may well wonder if life will ever be the same. That's asking for too much. How could life possibly be the same? First, by having a baby, you can look forward to a life filled with one of the most truly remarkable, profoundly moving, and perennially complicated gifts on earth. Second, you're just going to have to accept the fact that to be successful parents, you and your wife will have to reassess a great many of your priorities.

Rather than worrying about giving things up, look at it philosophically—from now on, your life will be expanding. Actually, your wife will be doing most of the initial expanding. (Prefather Warning: It's good for your wife to gain weight during pregnancy—not so good for you to do it, too.) But in less than nine months, your baby will arrive, and then your expectations will really start to grow.

Stop for a moment. Take a deep breath. If this whole pregnancy business scares you, remember, you're not alone. Prenatal panic overtakes most first-time pregnant fathers. Remember that your wife is experiencing the same anxieties. So this might be a good time for both of you to pamper each other. A gentle, caring touch always helps. Dinner at a special restaurant can also help, as can sitting together in the abundance of nature and realizing your connection with all life. This is a good time to begin filling your pregnancy with simple pleasures. And don't be alarmed if your pregnant wife looks at you with a slightly different twinkle in her eyes and regards you as her "prince charming." After all, the two of you have given yourselves one of the most cherished gifts on earth—the gift of life. So indulge her fantasies. Isn't it nice to be adored? Adore your wife right back. Remember, if it feels good to you, it will probably feel good to her, too.

You've probably also asked yourself a couple dozen times, "Am I really ready to be a parent?" Is anyone? The question rebounds through the minds of most pregnant fathers. The answer is, probably not. The reality is, however, if you waited until you were truly ready, you might never have kids. Rarely are two people ever completely prepared for the parenting experience they have procreated. That's one reason pregnancy lasts nine months. You'll have nine months for you and your wife to get ready to accept the child that will soon become an important part of your lives. That's three full seasons! A baseball season and a half. That should be plenty of time.

How you react to this forthcoming new lifestyle depends, of course, on how you see yourself in the world. Are you secure? Insecure? Confused? Terrified? Bewildered? Or maybe you're all of these. In trying to come to terms with some preconceived notions about themselves, some pregnant fathers immediately thrust themselves into intense therapy. "But I'm really still a boy myself. I mean, so what if I am thirty-two?" Or the really terrifying one, "What if I act like my parents? My kid will hate me."

A word of caution: Asking your father for advice at a time like this could be embarrassing for you both. "Well, son, you know when I was in your shoes, I just...You know. Well, to be honest, I never really gave it much thought. Besides, I was hoping for a Porsche."

The very worst thing you can do, of course, is to take your fears and frustrations out on your wife. She can't be blamed for your apprehensions. They're not her fault. The best thing to do is to tell her what you're experiencing—not to yell or to scold. And, as we mentioned, be prepared to listen to her fears, too, with a sympathetic ear. In fact, encourage her to air her fears, her hurts, her embarrassments. Tell her how grateful you are that she's carrying your child, and that you love her for it. Just a few warm, heartfelt words from you can help relieve many of her apprehensions. In a pampering way, kind words let her know that you want the best for her. Or, just listen. You don't have to have answers. You'll probably discover your wife's got as many misgivings as you do...and some that even put yours to shame.

We can't impress upon you too strongly that there are no small fears for a pregnant wife. Everything is BIG and life threatening to her. And her fears are real! So be prepared to go through "the unfounded worry period."

One pregnant father we spoke with said that from the moment his wife discovered she was pregnant, she spent the rest of her first trimester worrying about every conceivable— and some inconceivable—childhood disease she just knew their child would catch. "How are we ever going to cope with our child when she comes down with the mumps, scarlet fever, whooping cough, measles, small pox, colic, chicken pox, bubonic plague, and the jumping juju before she's two months old?" Which was quickly followed by, "My God, what about the teen years? What if our child is a delinquent; or worse, what if she wants to become a Hari Krishnite or ride a motorcycle?"

> HE: "We might have a boy."
> SHE: "A boy? But I want a girl!"
> HE: "No problem, dear. He'll be a girl."

One way you might handle these "real" concerns is, without being judgmental or critical, to coax your wife to write down all her worrisome fears on a piece of paper. Then, together, go outside and, in a safe and well-ventilated area, burn the sheet of paper and release all those bad vibes out into the air. It's amazing how good this could make her feel. You, too.

Although her fears have the potential to escalate into a chronicle of all the worst possible evils that could befall an unborn child, airing them is not unhealthy. And in the case of burning and releasing them, you do literally "air" them.

The absolutely wrong thing to say to your pregnant wife during her "unfounded worry periods" is, "Oh, don't be silly, dear. There's nothing to worry about." Guaranteed, she'll find a million more fears lurking in the dark recesses of her mind, if given half the chance. Better to cry with her, or commiserate with her. Never forget, a little empathy goes a long way. "I know there's lots to be afraid of, my love. All we can hope is that the baby gets our best genes."

What Happened to My Waistline?

A lthough we will discuss a pregnant wife's changing body in more detail in the Second Trimester section, one point bears mentioning now: Your pregnant wife will put on weight and add inches.

The first obvious outward physical sign of pregnancy is the loss of a waistline. Usually, at this betwixt and between period in her pregnancy, your wife can still just fit into her old clothes. It's also the time when she is caught up in a peculiar dichotomy. On the one hand, she can hardly wait to show the world she's really pregnant. On the other hand, she's not pregnant enough to look more than slightly overweight. (My wife didn't show until the sixth month. After seven-and-one-half months, my son, Ron, was born prematurely. My wife spent weeks feeling deprived. We laughingly referred to it as "The Immaculate Deception.")

Be prepared for those awkward moments during the first trimester, when your wife looks at herself in the mirror and her old clothes don't seem to fit quite right. At times like that a little sensitivity will be most welcome. Go to her, embrace her, rub her belly. Let her know how filled with wonder this process is and how much you love her. Never, ever, say to her, "Well, I guess we won't be seeing you wear those much longer," or "How's my little elephant?" or "My God, what have I done to your body?" Those "funny" comments not only won't get laughs, they're sure to do you in for the duration, and then some. Your "little elephant" won't forget those things.

The first trimester is still an adjustment period, when sensitivities are compounded. Joking comments will only multiply your wife's anxieties. Instead, try saying things like, "Well, looks like you get to buy a new wardrobe" (very popular with pregnant wives) or "That's our baby in there!" As we will point out in the next trimester, avoid all "fat" or "chubby" jokes, or be prepared to face some lean and lonely nights. Think lovingly. Speak kindly. Your wife will respond in form.

Weathering the Sudden Mood Shifts, or— Yes, Dear. I'm with You All the Way

One of the most unpredictable changes of early pregnancy is sudden mood shifts. Your wife might experience them up to the actual birthing process. It is imperative to learn how to ride out these rapid shifts in mental equilibrium. Realize that your wife is NOT RESPONSIBLE. We have heard stories about pregnant wives who have gone from laughter to tears in less than .05 nanoseconds (a nanosecond is equal to one-billionth of a second). One nanosecond, your wife may be totally content with herself and you, her loving husband. Then, whammo! Before the fall of the next nanosecond, she's suddenly berating you for being totally inconsiderate because you wouldn't eat the strawberry pie her mother baked for you six months earlier—even though strawberries make you break out in a rash.

We know it's the fault of those rambunctious hormones, don't we? So, when your wife is in the middle of one of her gut-wrenching 180-degree mood swings, it wouldn't hurt to take her in your arms and let her know, without being condescending or patronizing, that you feel bad that she's upset, that her happiness is important to you, and that you love her. When the storm has passed, she'll know that you know what she's going through, and she'll appreciate your concern. All it takes is a little love, consideration, and support. Love, consideration, and support. Love, consideration, and support. Trust us on this one.

That's the good news. The bad news is that pregnant wives can be unreasonable for what may seem to be no reason. So be prepared for any eventuality. Why do you think God invented presents?! They don't have to be lavish. You could give her a simple dandelion picked from the grass, or an "I love you" written on a note card. Then again, she may need more. If she does, go ahead, pamper her more. Indulge her. Maybe buy that expensive perfume she never planned to buy herself. After all, she IS carrying your child. It's a small price to pay to soothe the savage hormones.

Changing Lifestyles

"There's no way I'm gonna let this kid change my life." Face it, Dad, if you're planning to be a responsible, caring parent (and you probably wouldn't have read this far if you weren't), this kid has already changed your life. It's reasonable to assume, that in the few weeks you've known about your baby's existence, you have, in all probability, secretly painted glowing pictures in your mind about its upcoming life. You've sent it to the finest colleges, married it into a family of stature (if that's your goal), and seen it attain more success than you ever wished for yourself. Well, in order to give your child a shot at all of that, be prepared to make a few changes in your lifestyle. No pressure, but having

kids often means saying good-bye to some of your old imma-
ture and reckless ways (yours as well as your wife's).

Some changes should begin immediately! First of all,
your wife must know that pregnant women should not drink
alcohol, smoke cigarettes, or engage in the use of other recreational drugs. No two ways about it. And we can't be more
firm about this. The potential effects of such substances on the
unborn child can be truly devastating. A recent study on birth
defects attributed to alcohol-related problems called FAS
(Fetal Alcohol Syndrome) shows alcohol consumption during
pregnancy to be the leading cause of mental retardation in
babies and also of birth abnormalities such as Down's syndrome. Adding more fuel to the fire, a study by the University
of Minnesota reports that "Babies born to women who drink
alcohol during the last six months of pregnancy are ten times
more likely to develop leukemia during infancy." Researcher
Xiao-ou-Shu of the university said, "The study emphasizes
that pregnancy and alcohol should not be mixed." Don't try to
frighten your wife with this information. Just tell her how you
feel about it.

For some pregnant wives, giving up those harmful, but
enjoyable, social habits may require some special care and
attention from their husbands. Those wives may need a lot of
support. Giving up things you like isn't easy. So you have to
let your pregnant wife know you appreciate how hard it is for
her to give up those pleasures. But encourage her to make an
effort for the good of your child, and for your peace of mind.
On the reverse side, to help her ease the pain of her sacrifice,
your wife may ask, or expect, you to also give up your "evil
habits." ("Hey, wait a minute!")

So, what should you do about it? Well, it's true you're not
carrying the child. And you may find a dozen valid reasons to
not give up your "harmless" personal pleasures. You may
even rationalize to yourself, and to anyone willing to listen,

that giving up your pleasures would not be pampering your wife—it would be giving in to her. Right? Wrong! You have a mutual responsibility to bring a healthy child into this world. So consider changing some of your not-so-good habits...for nine months, at least.

Actually, abstaining might not be such a bad idea. It will cleanse your body and put off lung cancer for nine months if you're a smoker. Don't forget, even though she is carrying the baby, your secondhand smoke has been proven harmful to those who breathe it.

Curiously enough, most pregnant fathers we consulted actually wanted to quit drinking and smoking, and they found that their wife's pregnancy provided them with the excuse and motivation to do so. "I promised my wife I wouldn't while she's pregnant" is always acceptable. But if real differences exist—don't let them fester. Talk to your wife about them.

Your wife will have another lifestyle change that could suddenly impact your habits—more specifically, your eating habits. We have all heard stories about pregnant wives going through their pantries and throwing out all the sugar-frosted flakes, Macho Nachos, Twinkies, and Cheese Whiz, replacing them with hundreds-of-dollars-worth of health-food oat chips, granulated fiber bars, and dehydrated soy flakes. We will discuss eating properly and handling cravings in more detail later.

Remember, your wife's motivations are pure. She is only trying to do what is right for her and the baby. Pamper her by going along with her diet changes. Offer to pour her that bowl of dehydrated soy flakes with room-temperature soy milk. Encourage her to eat healthy foods. And then, when the opportunity presents itself, sneak a few Twinkies if you have to. This, too, shall pass.

Another profound lifestyle change should also be mentioned, even though you probably won't have to face it until after your baby has actually arrived. It has to do with your lost freedom to come and go as you please. During the first eighteen months of your baby's life (sometimes longer), going out to a movie or a restaurant with your little bundle of joy, and actually enjoying yourself, can be virtually impossible. But, if you're like most new parents, you'll hang in there and keep trying.

Take going to a restaurant. You may have noticed some parents doing the "parent stroll," and wondered what it was all about. If you haven't, watch someone with a baby at a restaurant. You will soon see one parent, then the other, wandering around the restaurant, baby on hip, desperately trying anything to keep the child from crying, screaming, squirming, or doing serious damage to the various leafy defenbachia. You can bet, too, that for every parent doing the "parent stroll," there are four others who didn't bring their child and who are spending most of their time worrying about the criminal record of their babysitter, and/or their child's general safety. The result is, new parents are rarely able to enjoy even the briefest of times away from their baby during those first months. So come to terms with this eventuality as early as possible in your pregnancy. There is little you can do about it, except go out to all your favorite restaurants now. See all the movies, plays, ballets, operas, and ball games (even pamperers need a break) while you're pregnant, because in less than nine months, you will discover the real reason God invented VCRs and take-out Chinese food.

An Unmentionable— Miscarriage

I n a perfect world, this discussion would be unnecessary. Unfortunately, we don't live in a perfect world. Miscarriages are a very real event, taking place in 20 to 33 percent of first pregnancies. It's more reassuring to tell you that 67 to 80 percent of pregnancies are safe and healthy. But if you go through a miscarriage, those statistics are not consoling.

Many miscarriages take place during the first trimester, without the pregnant couple ever knowing they were pregnant. For those who do know, whenever a miscarriage takes place, it's a tragedy. Just as the excitement of finding out you're pregnant is rising, and your pregnancy mode is in full swing, disaster strikes. Miscarriage is a painful loss. It is a time when your wife and you need each other's love, support, and consideration more than most other times in your life. Well-meaning, but seemingly insensitive or unthinking people will try to comfort you with, "Oh, you'll get pregnant again," or "I guess it just wasn't meant to be," or "Have you started trying again?" Often, they don't understand.

Laura and I lost our first pregnancy at the end of the first trimester. This loss is one of the saddest memories of my life. We shared our grief. We experienced it alone. We endured our disappointment. We did not take it out on each other.

From a physical standpoint, most miscarriages take place because something is wrong with the embryo or fetus. The body self-aborts. But according to the book *The Expectant Father,* more than 90 percent of couples who experience the pain of a miscarriage soon get pregnant again and have a healthy baby. We did—two.

Signs of a miscarriage can include abdominal pain,

bleeding, spotting (small amounts of blood), cramps, or all of the above. Don't hesitate to call your OB/GYN if you have a concern.

If you and your wife experience a miscarriage, your wife may not feel like being pampered. And you may not feel like pampering. But you have to be the one to provide some strength and sensitivity at this time. After a few days, the two of you might want to get away. Or, if that's not possible, stay at a hotel nearby. Have room service bring you breakfast. Healing takes time, for both of you. Then, after a few months, when your wife is ready, try again.

Laura needed about three months before she felt like trying to conceive again. A month later, we were pregnant with Johana. We told few people until we were safely into the second trimester.

More Changes

Although every pregnancy will inevitably bring about a slew of tremors that will shake the foundations of your normal modus operandi, pregnancy has a few quirks that you might not expect. A number of pregnant husbands reported that their wives began rising earlier and earlier in the morning. The husbands would wake up around 4:30 A.M. alone in bed and walk wearily out into the living room, only to find their wives chomping a bag of potato chips and mending a pile of shirts that were better-suited for the rag pile. If this happens to you, sit down, have a potato chip, and thank your considerate wife for doing such a good job on the shirts.

If you should ever awaken early to find your wife missing from her side of the bed, search for her very carefully. Whatever activity she has found to absorb herself will have focused all her concentration. Sneaking up on her could cause repercussions that may wake up the entire neighborhood. Gently begin calling her as you leave the bedroom. Give her plenty of notice that you're looking for her. Your other alternative, of course, is to just accept this irrational behavior, roll over, and get a good night's sleep. There's no need for you to get up, too, provided, of course, your wife doesn't insist you help her move some furniture or mow the lawn.

Another common pregnancy-induced manifestation is forgetfulness. Even the most organized of pregnant women tends to misplace almost everything she needs desperately. "Honey, have you seen my can of mace? And what's my diaphragm doing in the tool chest?" If misplacing things was a problem prior to pregnancy, good luck now.

This, too, will pass. Part of the forgetfulness is due to your wife's inner inklings of nesting. Although nesting tendencies will be covered in more detail in the Third Trimester section, many women begin them in the first.

You'll know your wife has begun nesting when you return home from work to find your house completely rearranged. During the early months, nesting tendencies seem to be fairly scattered throughout the house. Things that were in one location in the morning may be in an altogether different place at night. This pattern may continue until your wife finds the right spot for whatever it is she finds out of place. Often, things will be rearranged until they end up where they were in the first place. Your wife will be pleased if you tell her how much you love what she did, and that you think sleeping in the living room is a great idea. Complaining about it, or scolding her, will only arouse those hormones.

The difficulty, of course, is that so many things can get moved, even your wife may have trouble remembering where she put the TV Guide, or for that matter, the TV. As the pregnancy progresses, however, nesting tends to become more

BUYING PREGNANCY BOOKS **25**

concentrated in the new baby's room. While your wife builds her nest, you might as well try to enjoy the process, as in all probability you will be called upon to help with the moving. Just remember, it's your baby, too.

To Read or Not to Read? Buying Pregnancy Books

M y wife never found a pregnancy book she wouldn't buy, and your wife probably won't either. Publishers count on it. Our publisher counts on it, which is probably the reason you are reading this book. What pregnant fathers don't realize is that their wives usually expect them to have as much interest in reading these books as they do. Your wife will probably ask questions very logically: "Don't you want to know about your child? Don't you care?" You'll make points with her (and us!) if you say to her simply, "I do care, dear. I've been reading *How to Pamper Your Pregnant Wife,* which I find incredibly valuable to both our states of mind."(Gee, thanks!)

The main problem parents face when they buy and read all the different books out on the market is how to cope with all the contradictions. If each of these books offered the same advice, why would we need all those books? Ask your wife, and she will tell you she wants to have all the answers. We can guarantee one thing, no matter how much she reads, no book, not even this one, will ever prepare your wife for the fabulous experience of actually giving birth. But more about that in the Third Trimester section.

It *is* important for both of you to know exactly what is

happening inside your wife's body. Some time ago, the PBS program *NOVA* produced a profound special called the "Miracle of Life." It is still available in some video rental stores. By all means, get it if you can. The program follows a baby's development from the moment of conception through birth. Using the actual footage from inside the mother, the film documents the development of the zygote, the growth of the fertilized egg into the fetus, and then continues on through the fetus' growth progress. The film is beautifully done and is most informative.

Eating Properly

Y ou won't have to spoon-feed her, but your wife will know you're with her if you show genuine concern about what's good for her health—even if she doesn't always listen. The following is worth considering: A study published in the *New England Journal of Medicine* reported that women who began taking prenatal vitamins three months before pregnancy and who continued to take them during the first three months of pregnancy experienced far fewer incidents of birth defects and prenatal disease than those who took no vitamins. Check this out with your doctor. There's no sense in ignoring this information if vitamins can make a difference.

During the first trimester, morning sickness, evening sickness, and general hormonal overload might make your wife want to outlaw eating and opt for intravenous feedings. This is where you get to shine. In the most passionate, impressionable, loving voice you can muster, remind your wife that when she eats, the baby eats. And since you both want a happy, well-fed baby—and since only she can feed it—she has to eat. Even if it's a little at a time—grazing, we call it. Also, try to make sure your wife doesn't overdo drinks with caffeine or foods with additives and preservatives. Taken in excess these substances can be harmful to the fetus.

Remind your wife she needs lots of protein, too. It builds body tissue. Foods such as fish, meat, poultry, eggs, milk, cheese, and cereals made from whole grain are rich in protein. Milk and cheese are also good sources of calcium, needed for building strong bones. Leafy vegetables, liver, eggs, and potatoes are good sources of iron. Ask your obstetrician about a healthy diet. Also, you might want to pick up a copy of *Eating Expectantly*, by Bridget Swinney—a very helpful book on all aspects of nutrition during pregnancy.

And you'll be a hero if you assure your wife that this is one time in her life when she doesn't have to feel guilty about eating or be obsessed with her weight. And neither should you. Actually, most doctors suggest that a pregnant woman of normal weight can gain about twenty-five pounds. So let her eat cake.

Be prepared, however, as your wife eats for her and the baby, to soberly tolerate some various and bizarre cravings. Keep in mind that during pregnancy, your wife is not necessarily what she eats. I once discovered my wife sitting alone in the living room with a very obvious mischievous grin, and something obviously hidden behind her back. After a little coaxing, and a promise that I wouldn't laugh, she pulled out a half-eaten raw potato. Unfortunately, I thought it was hilarious and burst out laughing. Fortunately, the potato missed my head by a good foot, splattering on the wall behind me. Unfortunately, I had to clean up the mess between abundant apologies. Then we kissed and made up, and I assured her we would always have a supply of potatoes on hand.

Yes, pregnant wives get cravings. Yes, they are sometimes strange and unexplainable, and even embarrassing. One husband told us about his wife's sudden craving for milk,

which she couldn't tolerate before pregnancy. She also insisted on chugalugging an entire quart...right from the carton,
even when guests were present.

Another husband told us how his pregnant wife maintained she experienced no cravings during her pregnancy. Her
husband agreed, "Unless, of course," he said with a knowing
grin, "you count the five nights in a row we had caesar salad
with anchovies for dinner."

Another wife made her husband take her to a local super-
market because she had to have some Greek olives. By the time
this couple made it to the checkout stand to pay, the olives
were history. The wife sheepishly handed the empty contain-
er to the cashier, who deposited it with the discarded carrot
tops and rang up the sale without so much as cracking a smile.

Again, we must reiterate: Pamper your wife by going
along with her desires and the bizarre combinations of food
she must have... or die. But make sure she eats some healthy
foods, too. And if you have the stomach for it—partake of that
bacon-wrapped tofu and mint jelly with her. It's not bad.

Talking to the Baby

A s your wife's belly begins to expand (remember, no comments about the loss of waistline), you may find yourself
curiously drawn to speak to your wife's stomach. Many studies have pointed out that a child can hear in the womb, and
that children can be affected by what they hear. It should be
mentioned, however, that until your child has developed out
of the first trimester and is well into the second, it more than
likely won't hear a thing. But don't let that stop you from
making contact with your child. Talk to it. Go ahead, tell it
how you feel about it, what you're looking forward to, how

happy you are that it's gurgling away in there. And don't mumble. Speak out. Sing to it. Talk to it. This is part of the bonding process that your wife does constantly during her pregnancy. Notice her smile of approval when you do it.

Talking to the baby in utero, however, is not without its effect. We know of one musician father who, throughout his wife's pregnancy, played guitar and sang his favorite Irish song called "Maggie" over and over again to his then-blossoming son. Thinking he had to be close to be heard, this father sang directly into his wife's belly as though it were a microphone. It turned out this was not such a good idea. After the boy was born, every time he heard "Maggie," he started to wail and cry. With his second child, the father backed off a few feet from his wife, changed his tune occasionally, and was much more successful.

Sex and the Pregnant Wife

The good news is, yes, you can have sex with your pregnant wife! This can also be a special time for the two of you because, for one thing, you don't have to worry about using contraceptives. You can be as spontaneous as you want to be. The bad news is, during the first three months of pregnancy, your wife might not feel too much like making love. Not unusual. Often, all that is necessary is a little creative courting—and a willingness to be adventuresome and experimental.

If sex doesn't seem to be in the stars for you, well, look at it this way—you may just have to be patient for a little while and show consideration for your wife's inner turmoil.

Some of you may fear that making love will somehow

knock the baby loose. Virtually impossible! But if either you or your wife feels uncomfortable about making love because of this, you should talk to your OB/GYN. Neither of you should be shy about talking to the doctor about making love. It is, after all, what keeps OB/GYNs in business.

What can you do, Dad, when, night after night, your wife still doesn't feel like making love? "I just don't have the energy," she says. "Just hold me." By all means, hold her. Rub her belly and take heart, because before you decide that making love may have to be relegated to the back burner for nine months—HERE'S THE GOOD NEWS—know that an overwhelming number of pregnant wives report a heightened sexuality during the second trimester. We will talk more about that later on. For now, however, you may just have to settle for holding her, at least for a month or so.

A note about massages. After consulting our favorite aromatherapist, Tara Fellner, author of *Aromatherapy for You and Your Child*, we were informed that pregnant women should avoid some essential oils in the first trimester. These oils are anise, arnica, basil, clary sage, cypress, fennel, hyssop, jasmine, juniper, marjoram, mugwart, myrrh, oregano, pennyroyal, peppermint, rose, sage, thyme, and wintergreen. Fellner also recommended that those with a history of miscarriage should avoid lavender and chamomile, as well. Now, you may never encounter any of these essential oils on their own, but if you buy a blended massage oil, check the label. Remember, we're talking about oils here, not the herbs themselves. We will discuss oils in more depth in the Second Trimester section.

Congratulations! You've Made It through the First Trimester

If you've followed the spirit of this book so far, you've probably done some pretty nice things to let your wife know that you will stand by her through thick and thin—and that's not a fat joke. You've shown her sensitivity, and never ignored her concerns. But how do you feel about all the pampering you've done for your wife... and about yourself?

One pregnant father told us, confidentially, that he and his long-time buddy, whose wife was also pregnant, would get together and complain about all the things they seemed compelled to do for their wives. They knew from listening and talking to other people that they should be sensitive. But they wondered, "What's the big deal? Why the fuss? So she's pregnant! Why should that make any difference in the way a husband and wife act toward each other? And why should she expect it?" This father assured us he and his friend weren't insensitive louts, but he wondered, "Why do pregnant wives suddenly expect more of their husbands?"

For those of you who still think this sensitive approach is much ado about nothing, let's review what's been happening inside your wife's body during these first three months of pregnancy. Try to imagine the impact on a woman's system after that one in several-hundred-million on-rushing sperm plants its seed.

As the cellular multiplication process unfolds, and the zygote begins its magnificent transformation toward embryo, the hormonal floodgates are unleashed and the very foundations of your wife's body are shaken. This tiny embryonic cellular mass exponentially multiplies and multiplies again and again.

By the time the embryo is about two weeks old, it is approximately one-tenth of an inch long. In the fourth week, the eyes of your baby begin to form. In the fifth week, the nose begins to form. In the sixth week, your baby is one-half inch long. In the seventh week, it is three-quarters of an inch long. In the tenth to twelfth weeks, the embryo moves into the next stage of development—the fetus, and it's about two inches long. By the end of the first trimester, the fetus is three inches long and growing...and it looks like a baby. The organs are still developing, and those that have developed are operating at full speed.

While these changes are taking place inside your wife, her hormones are working overtime, keeping the process humming along at just the right tempo to produce your baby. It's like conducting an orchestra, when the musical piece goes from a quiet pianissimo to a wild crescendo.

That's what's going on inside your wife. And your love, consideration, support, sensitivity, and understanding can help her through the slide from awesome rumbling bass notes to trilling three-octave changes and back.

During this period most pregnant wives begin to experience fatigue, morning sickness, nausea, vomiting, swollen breasts, anxiety, and a general weakness. Some women experience heightened sexual interest; some, a complete lack of sexual desire. All these changes are not only tough on your wife, but on you, too. More than anything, your wife needs you to be there for her.

Understanding these changes may help you realize why she gets tired, restless, moody, inconsiderate, jumpy, angry, hungry, indifferent to you, super affectionate toward you, and sometimes willing to trade you in for a juicy hamburger. Admittedly, considering all that, showing compassion and sensitivity is not always easy. But you shouldn't be surprised that the little things you do to help her out, the insignificant accommodations—insignificant in the much larger sense—are appreciated beyond your wildest imagination. If your wife doesn't express her appreciation in words, she will show it through her actions. A very wise old Liverpool rock 'n' roll band once sang something to the effect that the love, consideration, and support you take is equal to the love, consideration, and support you make.

Congratulations, Dad! You've made it through the first trimester.

Keeping Her Happy

We randomly sought out a dozen pregnant women who were in their first trimester. We asked each of them to relate one special way their husbands pampered them that was particularly pleasing. Here are their answers:

- He bought me a beautiful ring when I became pregnant.
- Each month he sent me flowers on the anniversary of the date I became pregnant.
- He took on most of the dinner-cooking chores. He's becoming a better cook than I am.
- He phones me every day during his lunch hour.
- After dinner, he massages my back and feet.
- He helps me a lot with the housework.
- He won't let me do the laundry anymore.
- He takes me to my OB/GYN visits.

- He makes his own breakfast while I sleep in the morning.
- He takes me out to dinner a couple times a week, and often brings home take-out dinners.
- He takes over the children when he comes home from work.
- He tells me he loves me at least once a day.

SECOND TRIMESTER

Three months down, six to go. Before you know it, you'll be packing your bags for the trip to the hospital. You'll be turning down the home stretch. Oops, stretch is probably not the best word to use under these conditions. Better leave it with the trip to hospital. But there's no denying, you've got one-third of a pregnancy behind you, and the changes have already been significant, right?

But you can handle them. "I can do this. I can do this." Just remember, yours is the easy part in this process. Fortunately, in most cases, your wife and her body are starting to get the hang of this pregnancy, too. Well, your wife is at least adapting to the reality of constant change. And if she's been suffering through the first trimester with the morning heebeejeebees, you can offer her some solace by telling her she'll soon be able to...

Say Good-Bye to Morning Sickness

Yes, in most instances, morning sickness miraculously becomes a thing of the past at the onset of trimester two. That was certainly true for Laura and me. This is not to say that this is a hard-and-fast rule. In fact, we've heard about some women whose morning sickness didn't start until the second trimester. Then, of course some other pregnant wives we spoke to never experienced morning sickness at all. And then there were the ones who didn't know why it was called morning sickness, because they experienced nausea all day long. "I felt as though I was on a roller coaster, climbing and diving," one pregnant wife told us. As another described it, "I'd get hit by these sudden waves." And you can be sure she wasn't talking about a trip to the beach.

No man or woman knows of any way to avoid morning sickness. It happens. It's part of the process. If your wife's sickness continues, a sympathetic ear is all she may want from you. Cool compresses and a rose can be soothing. You might also suggest that she cut down on her intake of coffee and tea. Explain to her that they tend to be acid forming. Proposing that she eat a lot of small meals can be helpful, too. Saltines can only do so much, but grazing, eating small amounts on a regular basis, helped some women we spoke with settle the savage upset. Some vitamins also help relieve morning sickness. Ask your doctor or pharmacist about them. The only welcome thing to remember about morning sickness is, in most cases, by the beginning of month four, it leaves.

You're Not Fat, You're Pregnant

A s your wife enters the fourth month of pregnancy, she comes to a curious crossroad. At four months, she's not quite showing, but her clothes aren't quite fitting, either.

Back to eating. Although this may not make sense to a sound-thinking pregnant husband, encouraging your wife to eat during her pregnant months is a positive, pampering thing to do.

Your wife needs high-protein foods to sustain her and that life that's growing inside of her. She should avoid greasy foods as much as possible. Remember, snacking and eating small meals during the day is for her, not for you. You do not need to gain twenty-five pounds during the pregnancy. Remind your wife that she shouldn't feel guilty about eating.

Also, your wife should drink lots of fluids. Always keep plenty of milk in the refrigerator. Milk shakes, with or without ice cream, were a favorite in our house.

From the consideration file, keep a night-light burning in the bathroom and hall in case your wife wakes up in the middle of the night for a little late-night snack. Never forget, the better she feels, the less worry for you. And the added bonus is, she'll always remember and appreciate your concern. If you direct your conscious efforts in the manner we have been suggesting, we can guarantee that for years to come you will hear your wife recounting to other newly pregnant wives how wonderful, thoughtful, and understanding you were.

If your wife is particularly sensitive about her weight-gain, ease her concerns with kind reassurance. If you try not to notice her weight gain, she could think that you don't care or that you no longer consider her attractive. Simply assure her the added weight gives her more beauty, because it means something wonderful is happening to her...and to you. Call it "my baby weight," and let her know she can worry about it later.

During both of Laura's pregnancies, I found the tautness of her slowly expanding belly very sensual. Laura was one of those women that had a hard time gaining weight. Her over-eager metabolism ate up all those calories as soon as they were ingested. We had to do double duty on ice cream-laden milkshakes. She took these binges like a pro, too.

One husband we know who runs his own catering company began buying only organically fed and grown meats and vegetables for his wife. He wanted to make sure his wife did not have all those artificial hormones in her system. Of course, this led to what this couple refers to as the fifteen-dollar chicken. Proper eating is important for your wife. Going broke seeing to it is not a prerequisite. In this case, his wife had no trouble gaining weight. In spite of her husband's culinary abilities, her road to roundness was brought about by a pound of cream cheese and a loaf of bread for breakfast. Her husband made sure the bread was whole wheat.

The moral here is to make sure your wife knows that she doesn't have to feel any guilt about her waistline. We, of course, do not recommend uncontrolled and indiscriminate excess, which could be helpful to neither wife nor baby. We do suggest that if weight was not a problem for your wife prior to getting pregnant, it should not be one now. However, if you fear your wife has delved too far into the food bin, have your doctor deliver the news to her. Your job is to be supportive and helpful.

One final word on gaining weight. Understand that pregnant mothers who try to keep their weight down for vanity's sake may hurt their baby. Mothers who are too skinny have a tendency to produce unhealthy children. Mothers-to-be must eat plenty of healthy food. Every pregnant woman is different, as is every pregnancy. Make sure your wife's getting her share of proteins, nutrients, fats, carbohydrates, minerals, and vitamins, and you'll know your baby is, too.

In a time when studies tell us that fat is bad, we must not forget that fats are also an important source of energy, so try to see to it that your wife doesn't completely avoid fats. Essential fatty acids are good for her and the baby. So sneak her a little Ben and Jerry's when she's least expecting it. Again, the trick here, Dad, is for you not to eat everything your wife does. Sympathetic morning sickness is one thing; sympathetic weight gain is entirely another.

What to Wear?

I f your wife has been trying to wear her regular clothes, and has been letting them out when necessary, she may enjoy hearing these magic words: "Why don't we go out to buy you some new clothes?" I promise you, this shopping trip won't affect the college fund. You can reason with your wife that wearing maternity clothes carries a message, and you want the whole world to know how proud you are that she's pregnant.

My wife, Laura, is a used-clothes maven. She never met a thrift store or consignment shop she didn't like. Many of them carry maternity clothes. One couple we spoke with started having kids after their siblings and friends had children. They were lucky enough to become the beneficiaries of lots of hand-me-downs. Still, nothing will make more of an impression on your wife than taking her shopping for maternity clothes—not expecting her to do it herself, but going with her, and finding something that makes her feel attractive. A word of caution: As with most women's fashions, maternity clothes can be expensive. One husband's first response whenever his wife asked, "What do you think about this one," was always the same, "How much is it?"

Being aware of cost is important, but always remember love, support, and consideration. "It looks great on you. Knock-out. But do you think you really need an Adolpho gown for the office?"

It should be noted that some manufacturers of maternity clothes create designs that can be taken in to fit after pregnancy. You'll also find maternity shops have gone high fashion. Most of them now carry very attractive clothes for the pregnant woman—everything from jeans to party dresses to attractive skirts and dresses that have expandable panels to accommodate your wife's blossoming figure.

One sales clerk told us that many of her sales are to men who personally choose clothes for their wives. But mainly, this clerk found that wives come in with their husbands. So indulge your wife. And, then, don't forget to tell her how nice she looks in those new clothes. Pregnant wives often feel better when they feel they look better.

Helping Her through the Amniocentesis

If your wife is over thirty-five, her doctor may recommend an amniocenteses during the second trimester. Your OB/GYN may also recommend the procedure if your wife is spotting or bleeding. In the book *Pregnancy, Childbirth, and the Newborn,* written in conjunction with the Childbirth Education Association of Seattle, the authors note that the test is usually given between weeks thirteen and sixteen of the pregnancy. Watching your wife go through this procedure may be difficult for you, but she will appreciate your support and presence, even if it is in the waiting room.

When required, a local anesthetic is applied to the skin of the women's stomach, and a needle is passed through the abdomen and uterus into the amniotic sac. Fluid is then withdrawn and sent for analysis. This test is conducted with an ultrasound to make sure that the fetus, placenta, and umbilical cord are not damaged.

The amniocentesis tests for birth defects or chromosomal abnormalities such as Down syndrome or sickle cell anemia. For the most part this test is very safe, but it can cause some discomfort, and it is invasive. Any medical procedure that invades the system can cause a problem.

The fact is, women over the age of thirty-five have a 0.5 percent risk of having a fetus with a chromosomal problem. That means 99.5 percent won't. The old wives' tale about older women having troubled babies is false. Generally, older women are no more at risk than younger women for having a child with birth defects.

According to the book *The Twelve Months of Pregnancy,* by Barry Herman, M.D., and Susan K. Perry, M.A., Dr. Patricia A. Baird of the Department of Medical Genetics at the University of British Columbia conducted a study of nearly 27,000 cases of birth defects and found conclusively that older women are as likely to bear healthy children as younger women.

Of course, every rule always has exceptions, and for that reason pregnant women over the age of thirty-five are given special attention. The amniocentesis is invasive, but if a serious problem exists, appropriate steps can be taken early in the pregnancy with fewer complications. Let your wife know that you're sensitive to her concerns and fears. Don't downplay them because of the high success rate of the test.

When the test comes back in a few weeks, showing everything is fine, then your doctor asks the really tough question: "Do you want to know whether you're having a boy or a girl? Or maybe twins?" In addition to diagnosing problems, an amniocentesis reveals in certainty the child's sex...or sexes. Twins?! If you don't want to know the sex of your child, make sure you tell your doctor before receiving the results.

Another common but nonintrusive test we mentioned earlier is the ultrasound. A little conductive jelly is spread on your wife's belly, and a device that passes ultra-high-frequency sound waves is guided back and forth on top of the lubricant. Miraculously, on a tiny computer screen is the live-action image of your child in utero. Your baby is only four months old, but you can see its hands and feet, its spine forming, its heart beating. It is an amazing sight. Transforming. So, Dad, do not miss the first ultrasound your wife receives. It is a life moment to be shared like few others. Your first look at your baby! Realize, however, that five months from now—at birth—your baby will look much different.

The ultrasound is a diagnostic test and it is used to determine the health of the pregnancy. The doctor can see such things as whether the pregnancy is uterine or ectopic (in the fallopian tube rather than the uterus), whether all the organs are functioning and developing properly, and whether there is multiple pregnancy. An ultrasound is painless. So if all is well, you and your wife can watch the miracle taking place.

We should note that my wife, Laura, could never make out the ultrasound images. It may have been because she was looking at the ultrasound screen upside down and that skewed her vision.

Most ultrasound machines produce a printed image of the fetus, and some can even make a videotape for you to take home, but you might want to bring a camera in case yours doesn't.

Most of the time, prenatal testing gives both you and your wife piece of mind. But testing also provides time to handle the tough decisions that must be made should problems arise. Be sure that you present a strong arm for your wife to lean on during these times of stress. You should also know that you have the right to refuse these tests if you and your wife prefer.

In-Laws Don't Have to Be Out-Laws

C ast aside all those mother-in-law jokes. You're about to find out the true value of mothers-in-law. If you have one of those mother-in-law/son-in-law things (you know, "No matter how good he seems, he's never good enough for my daughter"), that relationship could change for the positive over the next few months.

Most of the pregnant husbands and wives we spoke to seemed to be absolutely thrilled about having their in-laws there when they needed them. And that seemed to be during and after the pregnancy. Consider this: Where else will you find more concerned, trustworthy, and loving support?

If your wife's relationship with her mother is good, then she has a ready source of invaluable information. Yes, things have changed somewhat since your mother-in-law gave birth to your wife, but the process is still the same. Being able to talk intimately to someone who has gone through it all before is incredibly helpful. However, if your wife's relationship with her mother is not very good, this might be a time to try to improve things, providing they really communicate.

In most cases, in-laws are not ogres. They're simply good fodder for jokes. They want the best for you, your wife, and the baby. You'll also find that most in-laws will abide by your rules. Of course, as we said before, every rule always has exceptions. Dysfunctional relationships do not heal overnight, so be prepared to do a little in-law pampering as well. Without anger, let your in-laws know, from a considerate and supportive place, how they can be of help. You'll be amazed at how well it works, now and later.

Be patient with the mother-in-law that has a tendency to

be overly protective and hovers over her pregnant daughter, wanting to make sure that she gets everything she needs the moment she needs it—and the father-in-law who immediately tries to take charge of the financial planning, preparing for prep schools and colleges the "child" would certainly be attending. Dealing with overinvolved in-laws is not easy, but you must realize they are expressing a desire and a need to be a part of this important event—the birth of their grandchild.

Actually, fathers-in-law are less likely to get emotionally involved in a daughter's pregnancy than mothers-in-law. According to a psychologist friend, traditionally, a mother has an instinctual attachment to the birth process. The father, while connected to his daughter, has learned through endless mother/daughter talks to which he was not privy, and then years of hearing, "Dad, I love you, but you don't understand about these women things," to provide a bit more distant support. Of course, some father/daughter relationships do not fit this mold, and as long as these relationships are healthy and functional, this time can also bring sons and fathers-in-law closer, as long as no hard-core jealousy issues exist between them.

In most cases, the in-law you'll see most will be of the mother variety. And if your mother-in-law is the clinging-to-her-daughter-when-she's-pregnant type, and it presents a problem, don't put it on your wife to cut the cord. Do it together. Talking always helps. Talking should help. Talking will sometimes help.

Simply tell your mother-in-law, in a considerate and supportive way, how you both are grateful for her concern, and how you both appreciate that you can depend on her presence when you need her, but that, right now, you have other needs. You'll just have to give it a chance to work itself out. If the situation doesn't improve, blaming your wife would be a mistake. It could be your mother, you know. Sometimes prayers help.

Telling the World You're Pregnant

D uring the second trimester, your lovely child-bearing wife will probably start showing (unless your wife is a tall woman, like my [Sam's] wife, who didn't show with Ron until her sixth month).

There's no hard-and-fast rule about when to tell people you're pregnant. Most couples have a hard time keeping the news to themselves, and with the first missed period, they start burning up the phone lines. Others tell parents early on, but wait until the second trimester to tell friends.

You'll find some of your friends will recognize the signs, and not say anything because they think you're trying to hide it. Some will come right out and ask, "Hey, are you two pregnant?"

But by the beginning of the fourth month, if all signs are "go," it's about time to tell. You could do it by phone; you could do it by sending out cards and announcing the coming event and day; you can do it by throwing a party for your friends and relatives; or you could do it by asking a friend to spread the news.

If your wife feels it's a sign of acceptance and affection on your part, then you do the bragging. Making an effort to be sensitive to your wife's desires when her body is in turmoil makes for a happier pregnancy all around.

The first time Laura was pregnant, I couldn't keep it to myself. Everyone knew as soon as it was confirmed. But we lost that pregnancy toward the beginning of the fourth month, as mentioned in the First Trimester section. This experience caused us to be a little bit more cautious about announcing our pregnancy the second time around. We may have been superstitious, but we wanted to make sure everything was fine before we told the world our exciting news. In pregnancy, superstition has always played a prominent role.

Folklore Is for Reading— Not Necessarily for Following

O ld wives' tales handed down through the ages have both glorified and vilified the state of pregnancy. Don't go for the one that says if you hold a newborn baby up in the air it will grow taller. It'll just cry more when you're doing it.

A lot of folklore concerning pregnancy was not just a matter of boiling water and hot towels. Much of it, passed on by word of mouth since early primitive cultures, concerned whatever seemed, at the time, to be best for the mother.

Folklore sometimes established taboos, rules, laws, and strange customs defining the responsibilities of the parties involved. Folklore about childbirth also spawned some strange superstitions—a few of which are still around today.

Unfortunately, in older days, outside of exhibiting concern, the father apparently had no other responsibility. Once the deed was done, having a baby was strictly the woman's business.

During the time of Henry VIII it was taboo for men to enter the birthing room until after the child was born.

According to Nancy Caldwell Sorel, in her book *Ever Since Eve,* among the Hudson Bay Eskimos, during childbirth, nobody was allowed to touch the pregnant woman.

Among the Egyptians, as far back as 1550 B.C., prescriptions for a speedy delivery included peppermint applied to the pregnant wife's bare posterior. Another was to plaster her abdomen with sea-salt, grain-of-wheat, and female reed.

Among the IK tribes in the Uganda mountain area, husbands were not allowed to enter the house for a week after birth.

In ancient Babylonian times, many women believed that the moon was the father of their child.

And remember reading romantic stories about how the American Indian woman would go out into the woods alone to bear her child, and her husband would wait in his teepee for her return with his baby? That's what was expected of him.

Some of Our Favorite Superstitions about Pregnancy

- If a pregnant wife carries big in front, the baby will be a girl. If she carries big in back the baby will be a boy.
- If a pregnant woman has a red streak down the middle of her stomach, she will give birth to twins.
- In England, it was deemed unlucky for a pregnant woman to take an oath in a court of justice.
- In Greece, it was thought that the fetus initiates labor when it is hungry.
- The Japanese have a superstition that if two pregnant women live in the same house one of the women will die in childbirth.

- Pregnant women of the Yukaghir Tribe in East Siberia believe that when they walk, they must kick stones and stumps out of their way to assure there will be no obstruction during delivery.
- Babies born to older parents are likely to be brilliant.
- Only males will be born to a woman who has her left ovary removed, and girls to one without a right ovary.
- Put a knife under the bed during labor, and it will cut the pain.
- If a door is open during childbirth, the labor will be easy.
- More geniuses are born during the month of February than any other month.
- For your friends who want to become pregnant: A woman who sits in a chair recently occupied by a pregnant woman will become pregnant.
- Prolonged use of contraceptives can make a man sterile.

We will supply more superstitions during the third trimester, so that you can know what to expect once your child is born.

Yesterday and Today

The romance of baby bearing, going back to biblical times, can't hold a candle to the tenderness of today's childbearing process. Not only are we able to take advantage of and enjoy the scientific and medical advances of the times, but today's pregnant fathers have more self-respect than their forefathers, whose wives had to rough it through the travails of pregnancy alone. So when somebody tells you it was less troublesome to become a father many years ago, tell them what yesterday's fathers missed—and try to do it within earshot of your pregnant wife.

Your great-great-grandfather's involvement in the birth of your great-grandfather was probably limited to impregnating your great-great-grandmother. Actually, not until the last few decades were fathers more than peripherally involved in the birthing process. That is, they were there, they offered support, they were concerned, but they sort of watched from a distance. They weren't nearly as intimately involved as today's fathers.

But that was then, and this is now. And now you can be a full-time participating partner to the glorious birth event, rather than just fertilizing the egg and then sitting on the sideline until the baby's born. Your involvement is much more loving, and caring, and rewarding. In deference to the fathers who came before you—it's not that they weren't sensitive to their pregnant wives' plight, they simply did what other fathers of the day did. Well, okay, they didn't know any better.

Naming the Baby

We'll touch on names during all the trimesters, but now, during the second trimester, when you talk to your wife's enlarging belly, all evidence points to the fact that your baby can actually hear you. And since some of you may already know your baby's sex, you may want to start calling your child by its name. If you have not yet decided upon a name, you've got your work cut out for you.

When Laura and I began to think about names, we recalled the advice of a friend of ours who had gone through this process a number of years before us. Whenever someone asked him what he and his wife were going to name their child, his was response was, "Either Fifi or Pierre." It stopped the asking.

We took this to heart, and whenever someone, such as Sam for instance, would ask, "So, what names are you thinking about?" we would reply, "Well we think the best name for the new millennium is Vinyl Spike. It can go either way, and it sums up what we have to look forward to." Needless to say, this upset Sam who, for a fleeting moment or weeks, actually thought we were serious. It did stop the questions. "Have you thought of a name? Have you thought of a name? You know, your great Uncle Aloysius, or your maiden Aunt Rufina..." Vinyl Spike worked for us, it can work for you, too.

When interviewing pregnant wives, we learned that most wives wanted the decision on the baby's name to be mutual. This is usually an emotional discussion, even though, as some wives told us, they were adamant from the beginning about the name they wanted. Since these wives didn't want to carry the guilt of their husband acquiescing just to please them, they listened to other suggestions. The women wanted the baby's name to be one that both they and their husband would love.

During this period, mutual love, support, and consideration are the keys to happiness. Laura and I had an agreement, if either of us said no to a name, it was taken off the list. It could be reintroduced later, but one negative vote was all that was needed to remove it. You want a name you'll both be satisfied with, and, of course, one your child will enjoy, too.

Where do you start? You can start by getting a pad (maybe a thick one) and a pencil and writing. Do it together. You both, surely, have probably harbored names you especially like, so talk about them.

Get the joke names out of the way first, then go on to the meaningful ones. Exotic names are usually a burden for a kid to carry, but, of course, it's your decision.

Make a game out of it. Take turns suggesting names. When you run out of names that come right to mind, try the phone book. You'll find millions of names in the phone book.

If you're star struck, check the movie sections in the papers. Or try book stores. You'll find volumes of books with volumes of names.

Our publisher, Meadowbrook Press, has a great baby name book with more than 30,000 entries. It's called *The Very Best Baby Names Book in the Whole Wide World*, by Bruce Lansky. If you can't find a name you like in Lansky's book, the name probably doesn't exist—but you can try your local bookstore, anyway. Bookstores usually have shelves full of baby name books—covering everything from funny names to religious names—whatever suits your fancy.

In the advertising business, which has been my (Sam's) business most of my adult life, we often conduct brain-storming sessions. These are sessions where the whole creative staff gets together and tries to come up with a great campaign idea or a name for a specific client's product. Every idea is fair game. Put-downs are not allowed. Often, we need a number of such sessions before our efforts pay off and we come up with something we all like.

The same applies to picking your baby's name. Agree on it! Love it! Don't settle! The whole trimester or the entire pregnancy may pass before you both decide on a name. That's okay, too. You may even ask your baby in utero to respond to names with a kick. One kick means yes, two kicks mean no. In the meantime, when you talk to your wife's belly, you can call your baby, "Baby."

Be prepared, also, for a multitude of name suggestions from your in-laws and friends. You'll find everyone wants to help—and everyone has a name for you—even though you might consider their help a hindrance. Naming the baby usually doesn't happen with the snap of a finger. So be patient with your wife while she's romancing with names. She'll remember your thoughtfulness.

After you've both agreed upon a name, you may not want

to share it with your friends and relatives until after your baby is born and named. That's a sure way to avoid any unpleasant or negative reaction—after the baby is born, no one will *not* like the name you have chosen (not to your face, at least!).

More Sex and the Pregnant Wife

S ex during Pregnancy? Outrageous! Fantastic! Cool! You're probably just a little, if not a lot, confused about whether to avoid or pursue sex during pregnancy. In ancient times, in many cultures, sex during pregnancy was a "no no." The answer was pretty clear-cut then. But we're not aware of any culture or religion where that is the case today. Now it's up to you, your wife, and your doctor.

We touched on it earlier in this book, but we consider sex during pregnancy an important subject. So read what the experts (and some who are not experts) have to say about it. This could make interesting bedtime reading.

In *Pregnant and Lovin' It,* by Lindsay R. Curtis, M.D., Mary K. Beard, M.D., and Yvonne Coroles, R.N., the authors write, "Intercourse during pregnancy is normal and even beneficial for both of you."

In *What to Expect When You're Expecting,* by Arlene Eisenberg, Heidi Eisenberg Murkoff, and Sandee Eisenberg Hathaway, R.N., in their section entitled "Switching from Procreational to Recreational Sex," the authors write, "For them, sex becomes fun for the first time in months, or even years."

According to Armin A. Brott and Jennifer Ash, in their book *The Expectant Father,* there's nothing to be afraid of. The baby is safely cushioned by its amniotic fluid-filled sac.

Unless your doctor says "no"...GO.

One couple with whom we spoke had different opinions about sex during pregnancy. The husband, obviously putting us on, told us that, "Once a trimester was enough for him." His wife told us that wasn't quite the case, as her sexual appetite had increased during pregnancy. She assured us that her husband never complained when they made love more than once a trimester.

One pregnant wife said she was very uncomfortable during the first part of her second trimester, and even experienced what she later discovered were psychologically induced pains. Her husband, she said, seemed to feel her pain with her, and they were content to just touch and hold each other in bed. Although this woman had strong sexual desires, and her husband knew there was nothing to fear, he patiently waited until she was ready. When she was finally ready, she became the pursuer in a big way. She swears she wore him out, and she was grateful he didn't turn away from her.

Another pregnant wife told us that she and her husband tried to get pregnant for some time, and sex seemed more of a chore than a pleasure—what with checking the calendar, and using thermometers and charts and such. But once she became pregnant, and she didn't have to think about contraceptives, sex during pregnancy became a more exciting and fun-filled experience than they had shared in years.

One pregnant couple we spoke with wanted us to be sure to tell our readers that "if they don't take full advantage of sex during pregnancy, they will miss out on the greatest, most sensuous, sexual experience of their lives!!" This couple said sex during pregnancy was better than when they were courting, because they didn't need any protection, and they had nothing to worry about. Sex during pregnancy freed their bodies as well as their minds. And this couple was looking forward with anticipation to their next pregnancy.

A few things that you don't have to worry about: You will not jar the baby loose. The baby cannot grab you. You cannot get anymore pregnant than you already are. If you still harbor doubts, here's what Dr. Stephen V. Lieb, Director of Women's Health Care Associates in Santa Monica, California, says:

> Sexual intercourse during pregnancy has been a controversial topic for both laymen and physicians alike. The opinions proffered by many a health care professional are based more often than not on anecdotes and myths rather than scientific fact. To no fault of their own, the dearth of scientific studies have made it difficult for physicians caring for pregnant women to render a uniform opinion.
>
> Women as well as their husbands will often enter into pregnancy with preconceived notions, such as: my friend or mother said that if we make love during pregnancy, I could experience a miscarriage, injure the baby, cause premature labor, give the baby germs, and so on and so forth. Sometimes it's the male who cannot make love to his pregnant wife because he feels ashamed to do "this" in "front" of the baby.
>
> In general, it is absolutely fine to engage in sexual intercourse during pregnancy up until approximately thirty-seven to thirty-eight weeks, after which there is a higher likelihood that lovemaking could lead to premature rupture of the membranes (breaking water before the onset of labor). This condition could then necessitate an induction of labor in order to obviate an infection of the baby while in utero.
>
> There are conditions, of course, where intercourse may be proscribed by the physician caring for the pregnant patient. For example, in a woman who has experienced one or more miscarriages during the first trimester, in a patient who has had unexplained

vaginal bleeding or bleeding secondary to a threatening or impending miscarriage, placenta previa (a condition in which the placenta is covering the opening
to the cervix), premature dilation of the cervix,
fibroid uterus, premature labor or prior history of,
premature rupture of the membranes, multiple gestation, etc. If a woman has any of the above, she should
consult her physician before attempting to make love.

If on the other hand the woman is having a per-
fectly normal pregnancy, there is no reason why she
should not continue to enjoy sexual intercourse
throughout most of pregnancy.

For Laura and myself, sex during pregnancy was a very
sensual experience. After oiling her round, hard belly to help
her skin stretch without scarring, other places needed oiling,
too. Of course, as the months progressed and Laura grew,
the main issue was always one of comfort. But the explo-
ration of different positions can also be fun, if pursued with
an open mind.

Unless your religion forbids it, sex during pregnancy is
not a no no. And as evidenced above, some pregnant wives
have voracious appetites for sex. Protection isn't necessary,
and you'll find your wife—if not making advances herself—
welcoming your advances whenever it suits your fancy.

And don't be surprised if your wife wants to make love
right up until the time she's ready to deliver. We have heard that
semen can actually help bring on labor in wives who are late.
An old husband's tale? Possibly. The point we're making here is
to enjoy yourself as long as it's comfortable and pleasing.

IMPERATIVE FACT: As Laura has told me over the years,
time and again, "There is more than one way to make love,
and they don't all include intercourse." If your wife is not
interested in sexual contact, don't pull out these pages and
point incredulously to the experiences of others. Be gentle,

kind, and compassionate. Being brutish or forceful can only make matters worse.

No, That's Not a Stretch Mark!

W ives are very sensitive about stretch marks. How can they not be? And just so you know (and make sure that your wife knows that you know), 99 percent of all women develop them. Stretch marks are caused by stretching of the skin through increase in weight and activity. Even active young girls of fifteen and sixteen develop them.

Even if you're sensitive enough to try not to notice them, stretch marks happen. It's part of the process. Your accepting attitude can help your wife overcome her concern.

Stretch marks can start showing anytime. One woman said that stretch marks first appeared on her stomach some time between five and seven months into her pregnancy. Her darling mother-in-law told her about a salve or ointment called Mother's Friend that she got at her pharmacy. The woman rubbed it on her lower stomach, where the marks first appeared, several times a day. She was told the ointment penetrates and adds elasticity to the skin and she said it really worked.

A variety of oils and balms are available, from Bagg Balm (used to soften and soothe the teats of cow udders) to vitamin E oil to aromatherapy oils and blends. Tara Fellner (our aromatherapist) has some second-trimester essential oil recommendations. In the second trimester use rose, rosemary, lavender, geranium, ginger, pink grapefruit, coriander, nutmeg, tangerine, mandarin, neroli, and ylang-ylang.

Neroli and mandarin are great for stretch-mark prevention, up to ten drops to an ounce of carrier (which should include evening primrose or rosehip seed oil).

Rose, benzoin, lavender, and blue chamomile are good tummy rubs, too. Fellner has told us, "Don't forget to rub stretch-mark-preventive oils on the backside of the body, too." More from Fellner during the Third Trimester.

As regards rubbing oil on your wife's body, this is your job. It's not a bad job, and it can be a very sensual job at that. It's also a great way to make daily contact with your wife... and your baby. You won't rub off the stretch marks that appear, but you'll certainly help so they won't become a problem. The oil rub will also make your wife feel good.

While you're oiling your wife's belly, you can also perform the pampering thing that outdoes all pampering things—massage. It's sensual. It's comforting. It's to die for. If you want to read about massaging, I recommend *Massage and Peaceful Pregnancy,* by Gordon Inkeles. The book is fully illustrated—it's sort of a basic massage for the whole body. For example, the book teaches that touching the body with soft strokes elicits a warm feeling.

Massage sends a message to your wife that you accept her fully, the way she is. It tells her you care for her. It shows that you are becoming familiar with her changing body, and caressing it with a loving passion.

Massage is an experience that can bring your wife closer to you. It transforms her apprehensions into a moment of joy that could bring out all her love for you, and lets you know that you're doing something that shows her that you truly care, and want to please her.

Massage is sensuous. It's as close to an orgasm as you both can experience without sex. It feels good. It is good. It's restful. You'll love it. She'll love it. We highly recommend it.

We have also been told that baths with bath oil and mineral oil help lessen stretch marks, and if your wife lies in the sun with her stomach exposed, her stretch marks could get lighter and fade. Laura tried sunning during our first pregnancy, and it seemed to work. Throughout the summer months, Laura would lie out in her bikini—yes, her bikini—and bake. Her dark, tanned belly looked great—very sexy. Of course, with all the concern about UV rays and skin cancer, make sure your tanning is done with a proper sun block.

Exercising Your Pregnant Wife

That's exercising, not exorcising!

Exercising during pregnancy is a YES. But strenuous exercises, such as sky-diving, skiing, mountain scaling, and scuba diving, are no, nos. Strenuous activities can be harmful to the fetus, so make sure your wife avoids them. However, you must encourage her to exercise. Check with your OB/GYN first. Unless your wife has preexisting physical problems or problems with her pregnancy, exercise during pregnancy is considered safe and healthy.

Your wife will feel better if, at times, you exercise with her. Pregnant fathers need exercise too. You can't go wrong with walking, bicycling, swimming, dancing (you can do that often), even tennis (you can play doubles), and, of course, your doctor will probably suggest some aerobic exercises.

Unless your OB/GYN puts your wife on a special exercise program, look into buying an exercise videotape for her. The videos are usually easy to follow, and they make exercising less lonely. Following are some of the videotapes that come well recommended:

Jane Fonda's *Pregnancy, Birth, and Recovery Workout*
Kathy Smith's *Pregnant Workout—Prenatal and Postnatal*
Denise Austin's *Pregnant Plus Workout*
New Bustles of Steel Pregnancy Workout

We knew a couple that took exercising seriously. Every night they'd make a large batch of buttered popcorn, pop in one of the exercise videos, and, while munching, exercise that hand to mouth routine as they watched the videos from start to finish.

One specific exercise that every woman must begin as early as possible in a pregnancy is Kegels. Also called a perineal squeeze, this exercise strengthens the pelvic muscles and improves the circulation to the perineum—that space between the vagina and the anus.

Why is this important? During pregnancy and delivery, the perineum is often torn or cut. The more supple and resilient it is, the better the chance for less tear. Also, the pelvic floor muscles support the uterus, your baby's gestation home.

Kegel exercises are simple. Your wife tightens the pelvic floor muscles—those muscles she would use to stop her flow of urine. She holds them tight for ten seconds to twenty seconds, and then lets go. The key here is repetition. Help your wife think Kegels all day long. We know of one husband who accomplished this by putting up stickies/Post-It-Notes all over the house with the word Kegel written on it. "Kegels, dear?" You're only thinking of her.

The Grazing Goes On

L et's give it a final shot. You've probably read all you care
to read about your wife's new eating habits. But let's face
it, it may seem to you as though your pregnant wife is eating
constantly. Actually, as we have mentioned, eating a little bit
at a time is not a bad way to nourish your child. And you just
gotta face it—her cravings for junk food and crazy food combinations are not about to stop. She'll stop when she's ready.

Many books on the market today explain a pregnant
wife's cravings for certain foods... but none of them tell why
it's that specific food she craves. So you can read those books
for laughs, but not to gain insight.

Do, however, try to discourage your wife from eating
foods that may require a swig of Maalox as a chaser—foods
such as salsa, hot peppers, hot dogs, sausage, bacon, alcohol,
and the like. That hot, spicy stuff will play havoc with your
wife's digestive system.

If your wife usually does most of the cooking, you can
offer to cook part of the time. It's a considerate gesture. The
meal doesn't have to be anything elaborate. The simplest
dishes often make the biggest impressions. She'll be thinking
of your thoughtfulness, not about what she's eating. Cooking
will also give you an opportunity to make sure your wife gets
palatable food that is also nourishing. Watch out for those
fifteen-dollar chickens, though.

And, remember, don't eliminate salt. According to the
book, *What Every Pregnant Woman Should Know,* by Gail
Sforza Brewer with Tom Brewer, M.D., "Pregnancy is one
condition in which the body requires more salt in order to
remain healthy."

Vitamins, as we mentioned earlier, are also important—
especially during pregnancy. A balanced diet will supply all

the vitamins your pregnant wife needs. But how many wives can balance their diet when they have cravings for foods they wouldn't eat under normal circumstances?

That's where you come in. Encouraging your wife to take the vitamins that will help her is not a full-time job. Just put them out for her. Little packets would be fine. Your doctor will tell you which vitamins and minerals your wife needs for a healthy pregnancy. You'll usually find she needs vitamins A, D, E, C, and B-complex vitamins, plus folic acid. Check with your doctor first.

Don't let the above scare you into thinking that you have to take charge of your wife's pregnancy. These are just suggestions on how you can participate in the pregnancy and voice an opinion. Your wife will know you're thinking of her welfare and that you want to help when you can. She'll appreciate your pampering, even if she doesn't thank you for it. Use this information as guidelines, not as rules.

You Deserve to Feel Good about Yourself

Congratulations! You just completed your second trimester of pregnancy. So what's been going on inside your wife's body during the second trimester? Let's bring you up to date. Once into its second trimester, at twelve weeks, the fetus can move around within the amniotic sac. By the sixteenth week, the fetus has grown to about six inches. By about the fifth month, the fetus looks human. Its arms, legs, and head have been fully developed, and it can suck and swallow.

Its heart is now beating away at about 120 to 160 beats per minute. By the end of the fifth month, the baby will be about eight to ten inches long and will be strong enough to be felt by its mother. Your wife should get a kick out of that. And you will too. Hair is beginning to grow on your baby's head by the end of the fifth month. Yes, it's a baby—a reason to be truly grateful. So far, consideration, support, and love have eased the stress for both you and your wife.

You can marvel as the fetus becomes active for a while and then rests. The baby generally becomes more active after your wife eats; she'll notice that. In the sixth month, all body parts of the baby are visible. The fetus is more than twelve inches long and weighs more than one-and-half pounds— depending on how fast it's growing.

Although still tiny, your baby is actually capable of surviving outside the womb by the end of the second trimester. Mother may not be too comfortable, but baby's doing great.

Keeping Her Happy

We randomly sought out a dozen pregnant women who were in their second trimester and asked each of them to tell us one special way their husbands pampered them that they particularly liked. Here are their answers:

- He takes complete charge of our two-year-old when he's home and on weekends, and he takes me to all my doctor's appointments.
- I've been sick quite a bit, and he takes care of the children and does all the shopping and cooking.
- He gives me wonderful massages.
- He indulges me with anything I want to eat, and sometimes he joins me.
- He bought an electric massager, and massages me every day. He's not judgmental.

- He's with me at all my doctor's appointments, and he does most of the housecleaning.
- He takes turns cooking and gives me wonderful massages.
- He props up my legs and rubs them every night.
- He kisses and hugs me a lot and kisses my stomach.
- When I don't feel well, he comes home from work.
- He holds my hand wherever we go, and he gets me whatever I want.
- He makes me breakfast every day. He does the laundry, too.

Of Course, I Still Love You

You're in your third trimester. It's safe to assume that by now your loving pregnant wife is blossoming into full bloom, and everyone around her thinks she looks wonderful. That is, everyone but your wife. She may be convinced that nobody wants to be seen with a bulging pregnant woman. She's miserable. She refuses to believe that you could ever love her again!

It happens. If it happens to you, you can't just laugh it off as nonsense. These feelings are very real to your wife. You have to let her know that you recognize that she's going through a period of frustration.

Many pregnant women experience this. Be sensitive to your wife's distress, but let her know you couldn't be happier with the way she looks now, and you couldn't love her more for it. Impress upon your wife that she's glowing with beauty. Show her works of master artists such as Rembrant, Botticelli, Reuben, Picasso, Jan van Eyck, Vermeer, and so many more, who found the remarkable transcendent beauty of pregnancy so moving they painted pregnant women into history.

Showing your wife the works of these masters tells her what she needs to know—that a masterpiece is at work in her. If that hasn't brought her out of her funk, take a bath with her...you know, one of those baths.

In the eyes of many observers, pregnant women really do

have a special glow. Besides painters, authors love to write about pregnant women. In Dan Greenburg's *Confessions of a Pregnant Father,* Greenburg writes about the time he saw his pregnant wife looking at her nude body in a mirror, and he couldn't resist telling her how beautiful she looked at that moment, and how much he loved her.

As mentioned in the Second Trimester section, Laura spent a good part of the summer—her second and early third trimesters—on the beach in her bikini. This is a story I have proudly told time and again. She radiated the beauty, wonder, and magnificence of pregnancy. And there was a lot to behold.

Your determination to set your wife's mind at ease about her appearance is nourishment to her. If you sense any negative feelings your wife may have about herself, you can assure her that pregnancy brings out a special beauty in her, and that you love her for it. Wrap your arms around her and hold her. Caress her. Rub her belly. Kiss her. Make love to her. She needs to hear kind, reassuring words from you. Tell her how beautiful she is. Then tell her again.

Building the Nest . . . Again

B y now, you certainly must realize that building the nest is a nine-month job for your tenacious wife. It started in the first trimester, and it's still going on. The closer the delivery date, the more determined your wife becomes to get everything in the right place.

This is a time to let go of any controlling attitudes or impulses you may possess. Let your wife change things. Don't try to have it your way. Think of the weight it takes off your shoulders—you don't have to make these decisions. Besides, the evolving state of your home can be fun. It's like putting together a puzzle that keeps changing while you're working on it. And just imagine how pleased your wife will be when you give her your approval and let go of the control.

Help your wife redecorate and move things around in the nursery or in the area that will belong to your baby. If you can't resist making suggestions, and your wife changes things your way, never say, "I told you so."

If you're an average pregnant couple, you and your wife are either planning to have or you've already had a baby shower within a month or two of your baby's due date. Unlike a wedding shower, this is a coed event.

Some enterprising friends of ours decided to recreate the game of Trivial Pursuit for babies. The game was incredibly clever, and we all howled playing it. I was surprised what a good party the shower was, especially when we began to open the incredibly useful presents from our friends.

If you really luck out, you may get enough baby gifts to stock two nurseries. Your baby may receive a changing table, a playpen, a car seat, a high chair, a baby walker, crib pads, changing bags, pampers, baby shirts, baby pants, snugglies, baby blankets, receiving blankets, and clothes, clothes, clothes. If your wife can wait, plan to do your baby shopping after the baby shower to avoid duplication.

When your wife is satisfied that everything is in its place (you can still expect a few more changes), it's time to take her shopping to buy a crib, mobiles, stick-ons, and posters for your baby's room—all the things that say, "This is our baby's room." It's a fun way to spend an afternoon, an opportunity to get out of the house together. Remember, your alone-time is shrinking.

If you know the gender of your baby, you may have settled already on the color of the room. A word of caution: In the book *Childbirth with Love,* by Dr. Niels H. Lauersen, the author advises you to hold off painting and decorating the baby's room until after your baby is home with you. His concern is that the paint fumes and chemicals used during painting may affect fetal development of the child your wife is carrying.

Although there is no sound foundation to Lauersen's theory, why take a chance? The good news is—it means painting the room just once, since your wife is likely to change her mind about the color at least once before the baby arrives. Now, that's a benefit.

But be prepared to move the crib, the hamper, the lights, and whatever can be moved, a few more times. Rearranging is good therapy for your wife, and it shows her that you are willing to make changes when the baby arrives. That's when you'll really learn about being open to change.

Another thing to be cautious about is your microwave oven. Again, there is no decisive research on the subject, but some OB/GYNs believe that the fetus may be sensitive to the effects of a microwave. So err on the side of caution. Offer to do the microwaving yourself, or insist that your wife not stand directly in front of the microwave while it's operating. Again, why take a chance? Or better yet, take your wife out to dinner more often. Enjoy it while you still have the opportunity.

Do Your Shopping Early

Y ou can't expect your child to get everything it needs at the baby shower. That's a good reason to take your wife out of the house to shop for those other necessities. As we continue to emphasize, make a day of it if she has the energy, and enjoy the time by yourselves. Below you'll find a partial list of things your baby will need, and you can take it from there.

baby oils and powders
baby towels
bathtub
bottles
breast pump
car seat
cloth diapers (useful for all kinds of things)
clothes, onesies, sweats
crib
crib pads
disposable diapers (if you decide to use them)
mattress
play pen
receiving blankets
snuggly
stroller
teddy bear

The car seat is important. You may want to read *Consumer Reports* on car seats for ideas. It's true, some of the best car seats are a little more expensive. So, if your wife questions the high price, tell her you'd be willing to give up a couple of golf games so that she can feel the baby is as safe as possible. That should make her feel good.

The crib is also important (maybe another golf game). You might want to talk with your doctor about your choices.

For other baby things, discuss your choices with some of the participants in your child-birthing class.

Getting Ready for the Birth—Take a Cleansing Breath

G etting ready means going to class. The third trimester is usually when pregnant couples go to classes designed to prepare them for the actual childbirth.

A number of popular classes are being taught. For example, Grantly Dick-Read is one of the first of the organized classes in preparation for childbirth. The Dick-Read approach involves prenatal education and relaxation techniques.

Another is the Bradley approach, developed by the American Robert Bradley, which stresses diet, exercise, and deep-breathing techniques. Bradley's preparation for childbirth technique usually starts in the first trimester.

The last, and what seems to be the most popular, birthing approach is the Lamaze method, developed by Dr. Fernand Lamaze. This approach includes stretching, relaxation, and conditioning, and the husband receives special training in how to "coach" a wife through the labor and delivery process.

Many hospitals and doctors also conduct their own childbirth classes.

In most of the approaches, the husband (known henceforth as "the coach," since at this stage of the process, he is basically a sideline influence whose job is to be a constant reminder to his wife to breathe properly and to focus during delivery) gets most of the attention.

If you can't make up your mind which course to attend, ask some friends who have been through the process. If none of your friends have had kids yet, ask questions of the class instructors.

All birthing classes are good. They all prepare you for the birthing event, and they all require you to be present when it happens. Your attendance at these classes means a lot to your wife.

You'll find the classes informative and exhilarating. You'll also be with other pregnant parents, which makes the process easier and provides someone with whom to share your stories. At class you'll be shown films of childbirth. You'll discuss exactly what's involved in the birthing process. You'll learn breathing exercises that you will do with your wife to help ease the pain associated with your baby's "coming out" party and to help your wife focus on something other than the pain. You'll also learn *effleurage,* a technique that uses light massage to help your wife relax during contractions. You'll learn about the three stages of pregnancy: labor, the birth of the baby, and the birth of the placenta; and about the three phases of those stages: latent, active, and transition. You'll learn about effacement, the thinning of the uterus wall, and dilation. You'll learn the various positions that your wife can use to make it through these various phases, and you'll probably see lots of films that are not exactly Academy Award quality, including films on delivery, breastfeeding, and cesarean births (more about that later).

Birthing classes are specifically designed to prepare you for your labor and delivery room activities, where you'll be (putting it mildly) the second most-important person in the room. While the doctors and nurses do their thing, you'll be the one to help your wife relax through the pain, to breathe properly during contractions, and to stroke her and massage her and be there. Her pain will be painful for you, too; but when it's all over, your wife will love you for your efforts.

Almost every book on childbirth has a section on birthing classes and approaches. The following titles are just a few of the books out there: *Pregnancy, Childbirth, and the Newborn,* by Simkin, Whalley, and Keppler; *Thank You, Dr. Lamaze,* by

Marjorie Karmel; *What to Expect When You're Expecting*, by Eisenberg, Murkoff, and Hathaway; *The Expectant Father*, by Brott and Ash; and *The Pregnancy Experience*, by Dr. Elizabeth M. Welan. There are many more, of course.

Your sensitive, supportive, and loving presence during your child's birth is of paramount importance to your wife. Helping your wife through labor and delivery, being there for her as completely as you can, is an experience that you will cherish throughout your relationship and life. Tell her that's why you're taking birthing classes, and that you are confident that together you will deliver your child, with a little help from your doctor. That's a bond that holds.

Laura and I attended Lamaze classes faithfully. Some fathers in the class didn't want to be there or were embarrassed by the whole exercise. And some wives were equally embarrassed.

Some of our friends had such positive experiences in their classes that they made birthing-class relationships that lasted for years. Ours was purely educational. We learned the techniques: how to breathe during the first stages of labor, during active labor, and during transition.

Taking a cleansing breath—a deep, releasing breath taken at the beginning and the end of all breathing techniques—became a mantra around our house. The words "cleansing breath" were the key to releasing whatever tensions were building. The idea is for your wife to choose a focal point—something upon which she can fix her gaze, such as a picture or photo. This allows her to take her mind off everything else except staring at the picture and breathing.

The important factor in this process is to practice every night. Not that we did that. But we did practice. We'd assume our favorite breathing position. I would sit with my back to the headboard of our bed, and Laura would put her back between my outstretched legs. We would take a cleansing breath together, then begin the various breathing patterns as I would gently rub her belly in rhythm to the breathing. We never once assumed this position in the labor/delivery room, but the breathing techniques we learned were invaluable to keep both of us focused on the extraordinary task at hand.

Practice is practice. It's never like the real thing. But don't ignore it. Use practice time to be close to your wife. Use it to develop your coaching style. Your wife will be counting on it, big time, when the day finally arrives.

Checking Out the Hospital

You can preregister at most hospitals up to two months in advance. Your wife will feel much more comfortable knowing that you made all the hospital arrangements well ahead of your delivery date, and you will, too. Check with your doctor too—your OB/GYN's office may be able to pre-register you.

Another reason for registering well ahead of time is that you will have to fill out a slew of forms in the admittance office. Patience is the key with these forms. Patience and a firm hand for signing everything.

Don't go to the hospital without your insurance card. Before you leave the office, beg them not to lose the forms. It rarely happens...except, maybe, in your case.

Before you register, inform the registrar in the admittance office that you want a tour of the birthing area, that you want to see what your room will look like, and that you want to know who will be allowed in the room.

Take a walk through the nursery, if they'll let you. Seeing

newborns is a great thrill to share.

Make sure you locate the elevators, so you'll know how to get where you're going, though you can count on hospital employees to direct you when you arrive ready to bear. Even though knowing every pathway into and out of the hospital is not essential, familiarizing yourself with the hospital can't hurt. You certainly don't want to get lost and wind up helping to deliver someone else's baby.

Make sure you're familiar with the parking area, also. Make sure you know which driveway to enter. It's possible that the hospital will allow you to drive right up to the door, or that it has special parking for delivering parents. If not, you may want to consider taking a cab. It's important that you understand that your wife will probably be very uncomfortable. And the less obstacles, the more she'll appreciate you. Simply tell your wife, as patiently and lovingly as you can, not to worry about a thing, that you will handle everything about getting her there.

Of course, you've chosen a hospital associated with your doctor, so that makes the hospital decision a little easier. But make sure you're happy with your choice—that you like the accommodations and arrangements.

Does the hospital have more than one ABC (alternate birthing center) room? These rooms look something akin to a room in your home, with lights on rheostats and tape decks for playing music. ABC rooms are available on a first-come, first-served basis. In case the ABC rooms will be full when you and your wife arrive at the hospital to have your baby, find out what alternative plans are provided.

Doctors often work out of more than one hospital. If your wife is not completely happy with your first choice, try another hospital. This is a decision both of you must make, but give your wife's preferences the greatest weight. She's the one who must feel comfortable.

Still More Sex and the Pregnant Wife

Even well into the third trimester, if the spirit is willing, you'll find your wife is more than ready for sex, and she instinctively knows whether her body can handle it.

There may, however, be exceptions. In *What to Expect When You're Expecting,* the authors address the subject of intercourse in the last weeks. They write, "Abstinence is often prescribed for women with a tendency toward preterm delivery."

In the book *Having a Baby,* the seven authors, Diana Bert, Katherine Dusay, Averil Haydock, Susan Keel, Mary Oei, Danielle Steel Traina, and Jan Yanehiro, all wrote of different sexual experiences during pregnancy—from no sex at all, to fear of harming the baby, to never losing interest in sex right up to the last days, to sex frequently into the last month. And we remember the pregnant wife who said she and her husband enjoyed sex until the day her water burst.

No matter what your fears are, those in the baby business say, "You can't hurt the baby." We've spoken to a few pregnant wives who were even afraid to take a bath for fear the water might harm the baby. If your wife is also afraid, tell her it's a scientific fact that when she bathes, water will not enter her vagina. Naturally, don't be ashamed to ask your doctor about any concerns your wife (or you) might have.

Of course, trying to find a comfortable position can present a problem. Experiment. Try lying in different positions until you find one that suits you. Try lying on your side...or putting your heads on opposite ends of the bed...or using a vibrator. Maybe your wife just feels like holding hands, or caressing you. Or she wants to be kissed or massaged. Pamper her desires. Do it her way. It'll be a pleasurable experience for you too.

However, if your wife is in the mood for sex, even if you aren't at the time, be sensitive to her wants. Who knows when the opportunity will present itself again? Just so you know, after your baby is born, your OB/GYN will probably suggest no sexual contact for six weeks. So keep that in mind.

From personal experience, fathers, waiting six weeks to resume your sexual relationship is taxing, but your understanding is absolutely necessary. Your wife needs time to heal.

Oftentimes, in order to make the baby's pathway to fresh air easier, the doctor will perform an episiotomy on your wife. A slice is made at the perineum, the area between the vagina and the anus. Discuss this procedure with your doctor. In fifty percent of births, an episiotomy is unnecessary. In many cases, the tears in the perineum that a woman may experience while giving birth may be smaller than an episiotomy. Be sure to talk about this.

If you have been sensitive to your wife's needs during pregnancy, you must also realize that the six-week recovery time after birth is important to follow. Waiting will be frustrating to you both. But as Laura has said to me, time and again, there are many ways to make love.

Getting Ready for the Trip to the Hospital

Since you never know when the green light will go on at home, signaling that it's time to make that dash for the hospital, make it a point to time your trip from home to the hospital before the moment of truth. It pays to do a few dry runs. Take different routes and try them at different hours of the day. When you gotta go, you gotta go—quickly.

Another good idea is to have a friend available to take over for you in case you're unavailable at the propitious moment and can't get home in time. In some cases, baby waits for no one. You can't imagine how relieved your wife will feel, knowing that you'll be well-prepared for any eventuality.

My wife and I had timed our trip to the hospital from three different routes and at three different times: during rush hour, in the afternoon, and in the evening. We could make it in twenty-five to thirty-five minutes, no matter what. What we hadn't accounted for was that our trip would take place at 2:00 A.M., on November 1, just as the bars were closing on Halloween. Talk about a spooky drive—thirty-two minutes.

The Birthing Choice— Whose Decision Is It?

N ow is the time to decide, as far as this decision goes, how your wife wants to have her baby delivered. Are you planning a natural birth, without drugs, with or without an epidural? Has your doctor predetermined a cesarean birth (a C-section)? Unfortunately, this decision is not always up to you and your wife.

A natural birth, without drugs or surgery, is always preferable because the baby receives no potentially dangerous drugs during its last moments in utero—remember, the baby is still connected to the mother. What mom gets, baby gets. But because complications sometimes arise—such as the baby being too big, or the pelvis being too small, or the baby being in a breech (feet-first) position, or the umbilical cord is prolapsed (wrapped around the child), or the pain is too severe for your wife, or because the doctor believes your wife isn't progressing through the birth process well or fast enough—a natural birth is not always possible, no matter how determined your wife may be.

Be sure all steps that *can* be taken *are* taken prior to drug inducement or surgery. And make sure your doctor is in on this determination. We had a hospital resident trying to make the decision about inducing labor when he thought my wife wasn't progressing fast enough. We demanded he get our doctor on the phone immediately, and he did.

If, however, your doctor believes the baby is truly in distress and all other possibilities have been exhausted, he or she may want to perform a cesarean. As mentioned earlier, know before getting into the delivery room what is your doctor's cesarean rate to natural-birth rate. If it's above 20 to 25 percent, question him or her about it. Doctors have been known to do cesareans because a natural birth doesn't fit their schedule. However, if your doctor believes the baby is really in distress or your wife's health is at stake, don't hesitate.

If a cesarean birth is called for, don't let your wife go to pieces. Calm her anxiety. Caress her lovingly and tell her that you both want what's best for your child, and that you'll be there with her all the way. After the surgical incision is made in the woman's abdomen, the baby is removed and the incision is immediately sewn up. Recovery time is longer—your wife has just had major surgery—but the procedure is as safe as surgery can be. That was not always the case. As late as the eighteenth century, cesareans often resulted in the death of the mother, because most doctors didn't have the medical technology to handle complications. The term cesarean comes from Julius Caesar who was a cesarean baby, and his mother lived through it. In 1990, 906,000 cesareans were performed. So much for cesarean trivia.

In many hospitals, you can be by your wife's side during the operation, screened from the procedure, if time permits. Under most circumstances, a casarean can be performed with a local anesthetic. For extremely rare emergencies in which time is of the absolute essence, the mother is put under with a general anesthetic. Whatever decision is made, if you can stay, stay. Help your wife through this, too.

Some pregnant wives decide they want their baby to be delivered at home—the way their grandmother did. If you have been working with a qualified midwife, and you live fairly close to a hospital (so if any complications arise you can make it there quickly), this is a viable option.

Laura's and my doctor thought that the only thing that should be delivered at home is a pizza. And even though many couples today have a well-deserved mistrust of hospitals, you want one close by if you need one.

If you live in the middle of nowhere, you might reconsider a home birth option. Discuss this with your wife. Let her know you're looking after her interests, and you want what she wants, but her safety and your child's safety should receive first consideration. A safe compromise may be an Alternative Birthing Center—these centers are not home, but they can approximate the experience of a home birth. Check out those in your area.

One common option for pain relief during birth is the epidural block. Epidurals are often given for cesarean deliveries. In the procedure, a needle with anesthesia is injected into the lumbar region of the back into the epidural space between the vertebrae. The anesthetic effectively blocks out pain to the abdomen, back, buttocks, perineum, and legs. One of the main problems with this form of anesthesia is that it can slow the labor process. Your wife won't feel the contractions, but things may take longer. She may also have less of an ability to push during the final stages of expulsion. This often means your wife will need an injection of Pitocin, a drug that artificially stimulates labor. An epidural may also necessitate the use of forceps or vacuum extraction to get the baby out of the birth canal. These invasive procedures have few long-term effects on the baby, outside of increasing the birth trauma.

A number of pregnant fathers we interviewed said they wanted what their wives wanted for the birthing choice. Most agreed that their wives felt relieved when they insisted that the final choice had to be what was best and safest for the mother. These husbands wanted everything done that could possibly be done to keep their wives as comfortable and safe as possible, and to bring a healthy baby into their world.

Be sure to let your wife know that she can change her mind in midstream. If she wants to try to have a natural birth and then finds she can't and wants to use an epidural, then let her. Support your wife's decision and never use it against her. You have no idea of the pain involved in giving birth.

Discussing Hospital Procedures with Your OB/GYN

The last few weeks before your baby is due will seem to last forever. Be sure you understand everything that's happening and what is expected of you. Make certain, on your last OB/GYN visit, that everything you should know and do during the birthing process is well-imbedded in your mind. You can expect your doctor to review all the hospital procedures with you. You'll find most doctors will patiently answer all your questions and allay your worries.

Yes, you also have a say in the procedures. Give your doctor—the hospital too, if necessary—a list of things you expect. Do you want an ABC room to make you and your wife feel more at home? Who can be in the delivery room? Do you want to cut the baby's umbilical cord? (Say yes, if you can.) Will you want to faint? Do you want to give the baby its first bath?

Make sure you are included in the birth process as much as possible. Find out about visiting hours. You want your wife to know that you won't leave her side for a second, that you'll be with her and protect her from the minute she enters the delivery room until she gives your baby its first meal.

Laura's birth option list was three pages long. Our doctor kept telling her that she had never gone through childbirth before and that she should wait to make the decisions regarding her demands. After that first baby, the doctor came back to Laura's bedside and acknowledged to her that she had gotten all her wishes and had come through marvelously.

The Last Weeks

B efore it's time for the blessed event to take place, how do you handle an anxious wife? "Delicately" is a good answer. It would help if you were a registered psychotherapist...or a student of psychology...or a guru. Actually, you'd probably have to be all three, and you could still come up with the wrong answer. But not to worry. Ask the average nine-month pregnant husband, and he'll shrug his shoulders and say to you, matter-of-factly, "Things work out." That may seem like somewhat of a cold answer, especially when you think about your wife, who's so tired of being pregnant that she could scream! But things do work themselves out.

Be prepared to accept the fact that during the third trimester your dear wife usually takes longer to do things... whatever they are. So have patience. Insist that she gets more rest and does less cooking. What an opportunity to experiment on some of those gourmet dishes you saw in one of your wife's cookbooks!

Remember, your wife needs to preserve her energy. One father we spoke to said, with tongue planted squarely in his cheek, that he felt the best way to pamper his wife at this stage of her pregnancy was to insist that she didn't take a second job. The point is, you should do all you can to see that your wife gets her rest.

One way to do this might be to give your wife nightly foot rubs. In their book, *Nature's Beauty Box,* Laura Sanderford and Amy Conway have an excellent recipe for "Poor Aching Feet Oil" from Southeast Asia. Mix together five tablespoons of sesame oil with six drops of clove oil. Shake and apply to feet. Massage in slowly. Now that's pampering.

Another wonder recipe—one that will relieve tension and puffiness around your wife's eyes—is a "Cucumber Eye Pack." To prepare this concoction, grate two teaspoons of fresh cucumber into two pieces of cheesecloth. Tie each cheesecloth into a little bag and place gently over each closed eye. Leave on for twenty minutes, then wash the eyes with cold water. If you do this for your wife while you're rubbing her feet, she'll be yours forever.

Learning How Far You Can Go from Your Wife

As your due date nears, you may begin to question "How far can I go?" if you have to be away from your wife. This is not to imply that you want to get away from your penned-in pregnant wife, but sometimes you may have to.

This can be a difficult situation. Both of you are well-deservedly on edge, and anything you say can set off a near-nuclear confrontation. This is not a time to let understanding take a back seat, but rather a period when your sensitivity to your wife's condition should be working overtime.

Granted, it's hard to do. Your wife probably goes to bed every night worrying out loud, "Am I going to have this baby, or what?" You can say very little to assure her that everything is going fine. Besides, you may be getting anxious and resentful yourself. It's natural. The truth of the matter is you may need time…a little time to yourself to get yourself together. Do you think a friendly poker game with the boys would help? That might not be a bad idea. Of course, while you're having fun, you can just visualize your wife pacing the floor, agonizing that she's about to have a baby and you run off to play cards with the boys. How could you?

That's exactly what happened with Laura and me. I went to a friend's house, who lives about five minutes from our house, for a gentleman's game of poker. The rules of the game have always been that we play from 6:00 P.M. to 10:00 P.M. The last hand was dealt at 10:00. After collecting my $1.75 in winnings, I proceeded home, entering the house at 10:15. Laura went ballistic. "How could you be so inconsiderate to be so late? You said you'd be home at ten."

She was two weeks from her due date. My first impulse was to laugh, but I had learned once before that laughter at times like these was dangerous. I took her into my arms, looked down at my feet feeling completely contrite, and said, "Bad puppy." She started to laugh, a signal that I could, too. She quickly realized she had overreacted, I quickly agreed, and the poker game entered pregnancy lore.

If your wife is afraid to have you leave her side, talk to her about it. Reassure her. We encountered many stories about wives' rising insecurities at such times. It makes sense. But if your sojourn is close at hand, and it's something you feel you must do to retain your sanity, without destroying the months of work you've already put in, do it.

Another solution is a beeper. If you don't have one, you might consider buying one or renting one for a short period of time. Just knowing that you're only a beep away can set your wife's mind at rest.

What's more, you must be patient, comforting, and reassuring when your wife calls you on your beeper to tell you she thinks she felt a contraction. And if she breaks out sobbing, for what may seem like no reason at all, remember, there is a reason— she's worried, she's unsure of herself, and she wants to jump out of her skin. So be sensitive and sympathetic to her emotional ups and downs and her frequent beeps. This is a very anxious time for her. She needs to be more understood than censored.

Tell your wife you hear her cries for empathy, and if it was practical, you'd carry the baby for her. You can tell her that you're scared stiff, too. We promise you, she'll feel better for that. After the baby is born you'll both admit you may have been a little silly. But now, the fear is very real. Talk to someone. Your priest, your pastor, your rabbi, your mullah, your psychologist. And talk to each other. These worries are real, and they should be aired and worked out.

Traveling Away from Home

I t's true, many a baby has been born on the back seat of a car.
But you've only read about that in newspapers. Very possibly, you'll find that going for a ride or a short trip will reju-
venate both you and your wife. Assure your wife she's not in
danger. If you're concerned about the safety of traveling during pregnancy, ask your doctor about it. Once the distance
and altitude are accounted for, your doctor will probably be
the first to say, "Get her out of the house...don't give up
living...the two of you should be enjoying yourselves." Of
course, you may have to stop on the road a few times so your
wife can go to the bathroom, but as long as she knows you
won't mind, a trip could relieve her of a lot of anxiety.

Then again, if your wife is too fearful to leave the house, it's
up to you to be sensitive about her fears and go along with her
feelings. Pick up a videotape of a good movie you haven't seen,
prepare a fancy dinner, or order a nice take-out dinner, and
make an evening of it. But if your wife can handle going out, it's
a great way to get away from the baby worries for a while.

If you have to travel out of town on business toward the
end of the pregnancy, plan ahead to have someone stay with
your wife, or arrange for her to stay with family members or
friends, and be sure to call her often. The tail end of a pregnancy is a trying time for a pregnant wife. For her peace of
mind, let her know that you have made arrangements to get
to her as quickly as possible if she shows signs of labor while
you're away. Better yet, if your wife is that close to her delivery date, consider changing your travel plans. The business
world is very accommodating to pregnant fathers these days.

You don't want to be the kind of husband we overheard

in our hospital triage who kept saying to his anxious wife, whose labor was progressing rather slowly, "You brought me home for this? I lost $2,000 at the convention because I had to come home, and now you're not having the baby?"

The doctors had told this woman it might be another twenty-four hours, because she was just in the first stages of labor. Her husband's disgust with her fears prompted this woman to order the doctors to induce labor. I had to hold Laura down on her triage bed to keep her from punching the guy. He was a lout. We could only imagine what was in store for that child.

Soothing the Anxious Wife

Make a personal commitment to be with your pregnant wife as much as possible during the last two weeks of pregnancy, and be completely available to her when she's close to delivery time. These are probably the most pampering things you can do for her.

This is also the time you might insist on taking over the household chores. Even some of the simplest jobs around the house can become difficult for your wife the last few days of pregnancy—whether it's wiping the refrigerator, taking the wash out of the washing machine, or brewing a pot of tea. Your wife will look to you for support—not only in a helping way, but emotionally, too.

This is an excellent time to take advantage of some "quality time" together. You don't have to do anything elaborate—just sit on the couch, cuddle, touch, and talk about what you both look forward to after the baby arrives. Also, remind your wife that you love her. (You can't overdo that one.) The two of you together…that's quality time. You know, once your baby is home, you'll be hard-pressed to find this kind of time alone.

Don't forget presents. They are always soothing. A nice touch would be to have flowers delivered to your wife when you're at the office. Or bring home a lot of things you think your baby will need. Your wife will like that better than things for her. Oh, yes, tell her, again, that you love her. She'll like that too. Remember massages.

More Superstitions

- A baby born feet first will have healing powers.
- A baby born with a large mouth will be a good singer.
- A baby born with open hands and fingers out-stretched will grow up prosperous.
- A baby born from a red water sac will possess great powers and double sight.
- A baby born with large ears will be generous, while a baby born with small ears will be stingy.
- At birth, a child should be brushed with a rabbit's foot to avert any possibility of accidents.
- A baby born on Sunday cannot be harmed by evil spirits.
- You can bring good luck to your birth child by spitting on it and rubbing lard over it.
- Beware, a baby born with teeth may grow up to be a vampire.
- However, if a tree is planted when the baby is born, the tree spirit will protect it.

The Night Before

Y ou never really know which is the night before you go to the hospital, so just pick one of the nights when your "ready-to-burst" pregnant wife says, "Tomorrow!" Then start packing. If you pack as you're rushing to the hospital, you'll forget half the things you want to take with you.

The coach's goody bag:

birthing-class syllabus
breath freshner
camera
change of clothes
Chapstick
coach's certificate
comfort items for labor—tennis ball, essential oils, diffuser
comfortable shoes
focal point
footsies
items for diversion—cards, art books, music tapes
LifeSavers/Charm Pop
lotion
nourishment for coach—easy to eat, nothing gross or disgusting
phone/address book and lots of change for the phone
powder/corn starch
watch with second hand
a little surprise for her

Some things she'll probably want:

attractive notebook and pen (to journal her memoirs)

books (reading is relaxing)

comfortable dress for leaving the hospital—pregnancy is over

hair brush and comb

her phone/address book

her toiletry bag (Hide a bottle of her favorite perfume in the bag.)

nightgown to wear during labor (if she wants to wear her own—it could get soiled)

portable tape player (Don't forget the tapes.)

pretty nightgown (for receiving guest after the birth)

socks and slippers or footsies (People get cold feet in hospitals.)

The best and easiest way to help your wife pack is to sit her in a chair, or on the bed, and ask her to tell you what she wants to take along; then you do the packing. Make sure you show her each thing she suggests before you pack it. After you've packed, set both your goody bag and your wife's suitcase at or near the door so you can grab them on the run.

Timing Contractions

When your wife's contractions start coming closer together, you'll spend most of the night with your stopwatch, keeping track of the time between contractions. You will also have to keep your wife calm—although most pregnant wives we spoke to seemed to be very calm at this point. The fathers were the ones who needed calming.

Delivery Dad's Obligations

Remain self-confident.
Keep your cool.
Give encouragement.
Provide physical and emotional support.
Be patient and understanding.
Use gentle commands.

While you're acting on this list, you'll also be massaging your wife's back, helping her breathe through her contractions, and trying to get some sleep. Help your wife use breathing exercises and focal point to ease the pain. Your doctor has already told you not to call until your wife's contractions are five minutes apart for an hour, which may take a while to reach.

Stay calm. If it is late at night and the contractions are still far apart, you might suggest to your wife that both of you try to get some sleep. She may not be able to, but you certainly can. This is not abandonment in time of stress. This is preparation for the work that will have to be done.

If you are unable to sleep, or it's the middle of the day, go through your lists, go over the route to hospital, and make sure you have all the papers you need, including your insurance card. Then, in your most reassuring voice, tell your wife to relax and not to worry, because you've taken care of everything you need for the hospital. Keep timing those contractions. Cleansing breath.

As Laura's contractions began, the night before our first child was born, we dutifully timed the distance between them and did our breathing exercises. We thought we were doing pretty well. Slowly the contraction time decreased— ten minutes apart, nine-and-one-half minutes apart, nine minutes, eight. Finally, the contractions got down to between five minutes and six minutes apart for an hour. We called our OB/GYN and said we were on our way. This was it.

When we got to the hospital, the contractions had fallen off to ten minutes apart. That was not the end of our ordeal. Our doctor came to check Laura and told us to go home. But before we could be released, our baby had to pass a reactive test—which meant that our baby had to provide evidence to those in attendance that everything was okay. Unfortunately, the baby decided this was nap time, and wouldn't respond.

Finally, eight hours later, after the hospital administered a tiny bit of Pitocin—an artificial equivalent to the octocin hormone a mother emits to start labor—the baby gave the requisite response and we were all released. However, we all returned the next night, when everything was really a go.

Three years later, with our second child, the same thing happened again. We had waited for the contractions to get to four minutes apart, only to have them drop off to eight when we arrived at the hospital. Our second child also wouldn't react. This time, instead of Pitocin, the hospital staff allowed us to use nipple stimulation, which releases the mother's natural octocin. We went into a private room, and I spent the next twenty minutes stimulating Laura's breasts. It proved to be a highly erotic interlude for both of us, and one that ultimately induced full labor.

The point of these stories is, don't be afraid or embarrassed to show up too early. You and your wife are excited, eager, and anxious. Many hospitals have pregnancy triage, where they assess your condition before you are admitted. You won't be the first to be sent home. Just hope your baby reacts more quickly than ours—unless of course, you get to try some nipple stimulation.

What's Been Going On inside Your Wife's Body during the Third Trimester?

In the seventh month, the fetus will be pretty well developed. It looks like a baby. It has grown to about fifteen inches, weighs about three pounds, and is starting to take up much of the room in the uterus. Its taste buds are getting keener. It can feel and even hear things that are going on outside—things such as music. It's also probably sucking its thumb by now.

In the eighth month, your baby will have grown to about eighteen inches and will weigh about five pounds. It will have moved into its head-down position, ready to greet the world. It can now open its eyes and can distinguish different voices.

By the end of the ninth month, your baby weighs about six to seven-and-a-half pounds and is about twenty inches long. Its knees are curled up, its head is down in the birth canal, its body will have completely filled the uterus, and it's ready to go to the hospital for labor and delivery.

Checking into the Hospital

Don't be alarmed if, when you arrive at the hospital with your wife for the delivery, the admittance office knows nothing about you. Control yourself. Hold onto your wife. They *will* find your papers and get you and your wife to the labor room in plenty of time. They always do.

Getting into Your Room

As mentioned earlier, many hospitals have triages for pregnancy patients. Instead of going directly into a labor room when you arrive, your wife will be checked first by a nurse or resident to make sure she's "a keeper." Usually your wife will have to be partially effaced and dilated before she'll be admitted.

Again, if you're sent home or sent off to walk around the mall until your wife is really ready, don't take it personally. Having a baby isn't something you do every day, and it's hard to know if you're as ready as you want to be. However, once the hospital determines to keep your wife, it's time to fasten your seat belts.

From triage, you and your wife will be taken to a labor room, where she will be comfortably ensconced—well, reasonably comfortably—until she has dilated to ten centimeters and is fully effaced. Make sure the labor room is what you and your wife requested. If you asked for an ABC room and one is available, don't accept anything else. As mentioned earlier, oftentimes those rooms are already occupied when you arrive at the hospital. If so, be patient and most hospitals will change your room as soon as possible. No matter what room you're in, set up your tape player and get some music going.

Tara Fellner (our favorite aromatherapist) suggests bringing your own diffuser so you can fill the room with an appropriate essential oil scent. If the hospital has caught on to the power of aromatherapy, you can prepare some back massage oils with clary, sage, and mandarin for a soothing uterine tonic, or a drop of neroli with tangerine for calming. Jasmine mixed with orange and a touch of frankincense is excellent for confidence-enhancing and will actually help your wife remember to breathe. Fellner also recommends a combination of rose and geranium to help create a warm and loving atmosphere to welcome the new life.

You can pick up essential oils at most natural food stores. Hey, I didn't believe it until I tried it. Aromatherapy works. Take the above steps and your wife will appreciate your ingenuity and your love. One note of caution: If the oil scents suddenly bother your wife, don't be upset. A woman's senses are on edge when in labor, and what works one minute may not work the next.

Once in the labor room, your wife will probably be attached to a fetal monitor. That's a machine that monitors the baby's heartbeat and your wife's contractions. You can decline the use of this machine if you want. We found it helpful in dealing with contractions, because the one we used had a scale line that detailed the intensity of the contractions. I could watch the contraction peak and let Laura know that "there's another contraction you'll never have again."

Stay near your wife for support. She may seem too involved to notice you—but she'll know you're there. This is also a time when you will be helping her with her breathing—

cleansing breath— and massaging her back to help relieve the pain, if she wants. Ask her if she wants anything—ice chips, a cool damp cloth—or if you can do anything else for her. When she enters active labor, the answer will probably be "NO!" but ask anyway.

We found that music was a great tension and stress release. We had half a dozen tapes, but it was a Bob Marley tape that seemed to make everyone happy—my wife, our nurse, the doctors passing by. Make this your experience, not the hospital's. The maternity ward is usually pretty lenient when it comes to the birth process. And as long as things progress normally, you and your wife should be able to dictate terms.

Going from latent labor to active labor is a real jump in intensity. This usually takes place once your wife's water breaks. This is when the amniotic sac your baby has been carried in bursts from the pressure of the contractions and the fluid pours out. After the sac breaks, the contractions start coming more rapidly, and your wife really needs to focus and breathe.

With our first child, Laura decided early on in the process that she wanted to look into my eyes as a focal point. It was an incredible experience. After fourteen hours, when our child was born, my eyes burned, but my love for and connection with Laura had never been deeper.

As the shift from active labor to transition labor takes place, and if your wife has chosen to give birth naturally without an epidural or other anesthetic block, you will never see your wife in more pain.

Don't lose it. Stay with her. Keep coaching her through the contractions. Be constant, loving, and supportive. Talk to her gently, calmly, without a rise in your emotion. Let your wife know you love her. Your job is to keep your emotions in check so you can be there for her.

So, What's Happening to My Wife?

The pain results as the baby's head is pushed down by the contractions, the cervix begins to efface (the walls of the uterus get thinner), and the cervix starts to dilate. The stronger the contractions, the more the baby is pushed into the birthing canal, and your wife begins to dilate.

Once full dilation is reached, your wife will enter the second stage of pregnancy—the birth of your child. We've heard stories about wives who screamed, grabbed onto their husbands, and yelled, "How could you do this to me?" or told their husbands not to touch them or they'd kill them, or called their husbands obscenities up and down the scale, but you gotta hang in. Just think about the pain she's experiencing and remain calm and constant.

By this time, you are either already in an ABC room or you are being moved into the delivery room. Your job is to keep your wife focused on her breathing. Pushing and expelling the baby is really hard work. Stay with her. When the doctor tells her to push, give your wife support. Hold her legs, if needed. Her only thought now is to get this watermelon out of her.

When the active stage of birth kicks in, all your wife will want to do is push. She will be instructed not to, as the doctor makes sure the baby can safely pass through the birth canal and your wife's vagina. This is often when a doctor decides to perform an episiotomy. This is the doctor's call, not yours.

Once the baby starts to crown (its head is at the opening of your wife's vagina), stay with her. With our second child, I nearly lost it at this point. I was completely overwhelmed with emotion when I saw the hair on my baby's head. Your wife needs you more than you need to be emotional.

The doctor will tell your wife not to push as the baby's head and shoulders clear the vagina. Keep your wife focused on her breathing, because she is just minutes away from being done. And with one final push or two, your baby will be born.

After looking at your child, quickly return to your wife's side and tell her you love her. Then, if you are to cut the umbilical cord, take a second to marvel at its beauty, its marble-like colors, and then do your job.

Now the "delivery" staff takes over. They'll immediately give your baby an APGAR test. This is standard operating procedure. It's a way to make sure that all the parts are functioning. The letters stand for Appearance, Pulse, Grimace, Activity, and Respiration. Each one is rated two points. A score of seven or better is considered good. This procedure is done twice. Your baby will also be cleaned, weighed, and given vitamin K shots and silver nitrate or erythromycin drops in its eyes to prevent eye infections. If you prefer, you can ask that these drops be delayed for an hour so that your baby can see clearly for a while.

Just when you thought your job was over, one more thing needs to be done—the final stage of birth, the birth of the placenta. This normally takes place ten to twenty minutes after the baby is born. The expulsion may require some added breathing for the contractions that follow, but in most cases, mother and father are so engrossed with their newborn baby, that the birth of the placenta—the organ that protected your baby for nine months—is hardly noticed.

A side note: If you have the stomach for such things, take a look at the placenta before it's sent off for testing. It's quite an amazing-looking thing.

Keeping Her Happy

We randomly sought out a dozen pregnant women who were in their third trimester. We asked each of them to relate one special way their husbands pampered them that was particularly pleasing. Here are their answers:

- I had to stay in bed during the entire last three months of my pregnancy, so my husband did everything for me. I was really pampered.
- He told me to call him at his office if I needed anything at all and he would take care of it…and he did!
- He let me wear his shirts.
- He brought me breakfast in bed every day.
- He was very supportive. He insisted that I not work during the third trimester. It really made me feel good.
- He took me on a cruise and we spent eight days together. I didn't have to lift a finger.
- He arranged to have his parents (my in-laws) take the children the last month. It was like a second honeymoon.
- Whenever I had an instant craving for a hamburger, he'd immediately take me to the closest burger joint he could find. And he seemed to know where they all were.
- He was constantly supportive. He made sure I always took my nap.
- He would listen to me even when I was cranky.
- He's a very regimented guy, and he let go of his schedules and was willing to let me take my time.
- He would see to the dirty dishes and cleaning without being asked.

You Made It, Didn't You?

We're convinced if you did all the pampering things suggested in this book, you'll be up for sainthood. So do those you're comfortable with, and for your wife's sake, try the others. We hope you will make a sincere attempt to be sensitive and supportive to your wife's condition, and we hope you now realize that your pregnant wife needs and deserves pampering through these most-difficult and heartwarming nine months.

All our interviews testify overwhelmingly that the whole nine-month saga is worth every sacrifice made, especially so when, within a day or so after your beautiful baby's birth, you will take your child home with you.

My wife and I (Sam) didn't get to experience that euphoria with Ron. As I mentioned earlier, Ron was born six weeks premature. He was kept in the hospital for a couple of weeks before we could take him home. I envy all of you who did experience it.

Laura and I did experience that joy. In fact, my father and mother and sister and brother-in-law were in the delivery room ten minutes after the baby was born, seeing their grandchild and niece in all her beauty. What a day!

When you look back on it, we promise you'll also agree the pregnancy was a wonderful, growing experience. And look what you had to look forward to—a new, exciting adventure in your life, complete with laughter, tears, love, and compassion.

No matter what goals you reach in the future, your pregnancy will invariably be one of the highlights of your life, and, without question, one of the best things you'll ever do. Enjoy it. Enjoy the new life you bring into your home. And, oh, yes, give our regards to your wife.

——————**THE BEGINNING**——————

LETTER FROM A PAMPERED WIFE

January 1997
Santa Fe, New Mexico

Dear Reader,

When Ron and I first decided it was time to have a child, it was both thrilling and terrifying. A pregnancy can be a very conflicted time for a woman. The loss of body shape, the giving up of freedoms, and the changes it can bring to a relationship all weigh heavily on the mind. I know, I went through many nights worrying about all of these issues.

However, I was very fortunate in many ways. Ron was at my side to help me through my ups and downs, rubbed my stomach with vitamin E oils to prevent stretch marks, and made me feel loved and appreciated no matter what my weight was. He cooked every meal, helped me clean the house, and never complained about what I might say, do, or want to eat (except when I swore that once the baby was born I was going to buy a Harley and shave my head). The truth is, he actually did many of the things described in this book and he survived to write about it.

As Ron and Sam made clear, the long time it takes for a baby to develop is a blessing. It is the time to work together to establish a bond with each other that will help in the transition when the baby finally comes. A woman needs support, love, and consideration from her mate during this time. Ron gave me all of those things and I was very grateful. His charming companionship, his humor, his tender care, and his wonderful pampering of me made my pregnancy and birth a miraculous event filled with great joy and happiness. I wish you the same joy. I also hope you can find in this book the support and encouragement you need to experience something similar with your wife. From one who's been there, the results will be worth your effort.

Sincerely yours,

Laura Sanderford

BIBLIOGRAPHY

Atalla, Bill M., with Steve Beitler. *The Thirteen Months of Pregnancy*. St. Helena, California: Oddly Enough, 1992.

Bert, Diana; Kathrine Dusay; Avril Haydock; Susan Keel; Mary Oei; Danielle Steel Traina; and Jan Yanehiro. *Having a Baby*. New York: Dell, 1980.

Bittman, Sam, and Sue Rosenberg Zalk. *Expectant Fathers*. New York: Ballentine Books, 1978.

Bratton, Fred Gladstone. *Myths and Legends of the Ancient Near East*. New York: Thomas Y. Crowell Co., 1970.

Brewer, Gail Sforza, with Tom Brewer, M.D. *What Every Pregnant Woman Should Know*. New York: Random House, 1977.

Brott, Armin A., and Jennifer Ash. *The Expectant Father*. New York: Abbeville Publishing Group, 1995.

Chamberlain, Alexander Francis. *The Child and Childhood in Folk-Thought*. New York and London: Macmillan and Co., 1896.

Chamberlain, Mary. *Old Wives' Tales*. London: Virago Press, 1981.

Coffin, Tristram P., and Hennig Cohen. *Folklore in America*. New York: Doubleday & Company, 1966.

Curtis, Lindsay R., M.D.; Mary K. Beard, M.D.; and Yvonne Coroles. *Pregnant and Lovin' It*. New York: The Body Press, 1992.

Eisenberg, Arlene; Heidi Eisenberg; and Sandy Eisenberg Hathaway. *What to Expect When You're Expecting.* New York: Workman Publishing, 1984.

Greenburg, Dan. *Confessions of a Pregnant Father.* New York: Ballentine Books, 1987.

Hallen, Mark. *Don't Mind Him He's Pregnant.* Berkeley: Ten Speed Press, 1984.

Herman, Barry, M.D., and Susan K. Perry. *The Twelve-Month Pregnancy.* Los Angeles: Lowell House, 1992.

Hill, Thomas. *What to Expect When Your Wife is Expanding.* New York: Cader Books, 1993.

Inkeles, Gordon. *Massage and Peaceful Pregnancy.* New York: Perigee Books, Putnam Publishing, 1983.

Kallop, Fritzi Farber, with Julie Houston. *Fritzi Kallop's Birth Book.* New York: Vintage Books, 1988.

Karmel, Marjorie. *Thank You, Dr. Lamaze.* New York: Harper Colophon Books, 1959.

Lansky, Bruce. *The Very Best Baby Name Book in the Whole Wide World.* Deephaven: Meadowbrook Press, 1995.

Lauersen, Dr. Niels H. *Childbirth with Love.* New York: G.P. Putnam's Sons, 1983.

Morales, Karla, and Charles B. Inlander. *Take This Book to the Obstetrician with You.* Reading: Addison-Wesley Publishing, 1991.

New England Journal of Medicine. Boston: Boston Massachusetts Medical Society. January 1989.

Opie, Iona, and Moria Tatem. *A Dictionary of Superstitions.* New York: Oxford University Press, 1989.

Rob, Caroline, editor. *Glamour Guide to Pregnancy.* New York: Fawcett Columbine, 1986.

Russell, Keith P., M.D., and Jennifer Niebyl, M.D. *Eastman's Expectant Motherhood.* Canada: Little, Brown & Company, 1989.

Sanderford, Laura, and Amy Conway. *Nature's Beauty Box.* Boston: Charles Tuttle, 1995.

Sarnott, Tane, and Reynold Ruffins. *Take Warning!* New York: Charles Scribner's Sons, 1978.

Simkin, Penny; Janet Whalley; and Ann Keppler. *Pregnancy, Childbirth, and the Newborn.* Deephaven: Meadowbrook Press, 1991.

Sorel, Nancy Caldwell. *Ever Since Eve.* New York: Oxford University Press, 1984.

Stautbert, Susan Schiffer. *Pregnancy Nine to Five.* New York: Simon & Schuster, 1985.

Strom, Charles M., M.D. *Have a Healthy Baby.* New York: Prentice Hall, 1988.

Swinney, Bridget. *Eating Expectantly.* Deephaven: Meadowbrook Press, 1996.

Walker, Morton; Bernice Yoffee; and Park H. Gray, M.D. *The Complete Book of Birth.* New York: Simon & Schuster, 1979.

Whelan, Dr. Elizabeth M. *The Pregnancy Experience.* New York: W.W. Norton, 1978.

Order Form

Qty.	Title	Author	Order No.	Unit Cost (U.S. $)	Total
	Baby & Child Emergency First Aid	Einzig, M.	1380	$15.00	
	Baby & Child Medical Care	Hart, T.	1159	$9.00	
	Baby Journal	Bennett, M.	3172	$10.00	
	Baby Name Personality Survey	Lansky/Sinrod	1270	$8.00	
	Best Baby Shower Book	Cooke, C.	1239	$7.00	
	Child Care A to Z	Woolfson, R.	1010	$13.00	
	Discipline without Shouting or Spanking	Wyckoff/Unell	1079	$6.00	
	Eating Expectantly	Swinney, B.	1135	$12.00	
	Familiarity Breeds Children	Lansky, B.	4015	$7.00	
	Feed Me! I'm Yours	Lansky, V.	1109	$9.00	
	Gentle Discipline	Lighter, D.	1085	$6.00	
	Getting Organized for Your New Baby	Bard, M.	1229	$9.00	
	Grandma Knows Best	McBride, M.	4009	$7.00	
	Hi, Mom! Hi, Dad!	Johnston, L.	1139	$6.00	
	Joy of Parenthood	Blaustone, J.	3500	$6.00	
	Maternal Journal	Bennett, M.	3171	$10.00	
	Practical Parenting Tips	Lansky, V.	1180	$8.00	
	Pregnancy, Childbirth, and the Newborn	Simkin/Whalley/Keppler	1169	$12.00	
	Very Best Baby Name Book	Lansky, B.	1030	$8.00	
				Subtotal	
			Shipping and Handling (see below)		
			MN residents add 6.5% sales tax		
				Total	

YES! Please send me the books indicated above. Add $2.00 shipping and handling for the first book and 50¢ for each additional book. Add $2.50 to total for books shipped to Canada. Overseas postage will be billed. Allow up to four weeks for delivery. Send check or money order payable to Meadowbrook Press. No cash or C.O.D.'s, please. Prices subject to change without notice. **Quantity discounts available upon request.**

Send book(s) to:

Name _____

Address _____

City _____ State _____ Zip _____

Telephone (_____)_____

Purchase order number (if necessary) _____

Payment via:

☐ Check or money order payable to Meadowbrook Press (No cash or C.O.D.'s, please.)

Amount enclosed $ _____

☐ Visa (for orders over $10.00 only)   ☐ MasterCard (for orders over $10.00 only)

Account #_____

Signature _____ Exp. Date_____

A **FREE** Meadowbrook catalog is available upon request.
You can also phone us for orders of $10.00 or more at 1-800-338-2232.

Mail to: Meadowbrook Press
5451 Smetana Drive, Minnetonka, Minnesota 55343

Phone (612) 930-1100   Toll-Free 1-800-338-2232   Fax (612) 930-1940